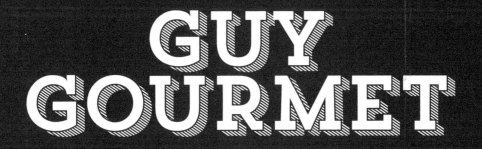

GUY GOURMET

GUY GOURMET

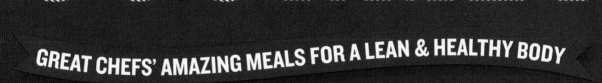

GREAT CHEFS' AMAZING MEALS FOR A LEAN & HEALTHY BODY

Adina Steiman & *Paul Kita*
with the editors of

MensHealth

photographs by
Jennifer May

Book design by Mike Smith

Photographs by Jennifer May

except Thomas McDonald/Rodale Images: pages 9, 11 (thermometer), 78, 154-155; Thomas McDonald/
Mitch Mandel/Rodale Images: pages 10, 11 (spoon), 12 (slow cooker), 207; photodisc: page 11 (measuring spoons);
Mitch Mandel/Rodale Images: page 12 (cutting board); Arco images GmbH/Alamy: page 73 (popcorn);
Mike Smith: page 73; Levi Brown: page 175

Food styling by Paul Grimes; prop styling by Barb Fritz

Illustrations by Jameson Simpson

Library of Congress Cataloging-in-Publication Data is on file with the publisher.

ISBN 978-1-60961-980-0   direct hardcover
ISBN 978-1-60961-979-4   trade hardcover

Distributed to the trade by Macmillan

2 4 6 8 10 9 7 5 3   direct hardcover
2 4 6 8 10 9 7 5 3   trade hardcover

We inspire and enable people to improve their lives and the world around them.
www.rodalebooks.com

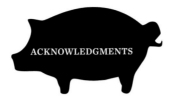

ACKNOWLEDGMENTS

Years of hard work by *Men's Health* editors, researchers, recipe developers, and writers gave us a wealth of material to choose from for this collection. Thanks to all of them, especially former food and nutrition editor Matt Goulding and the always hungry Peter Moore. On this project, we relied on the editorial insight, patience, and deep institutional knowledge of our book editor, Jeff Csatari. George Karabotsos and Mike Smith gave the book its brilliant design. Our thanks go out to project editors Erin Williams and Hope Clarke and the team at Rodale Books, including Beth Lamb, Brent Gallenberger, Sara Cox, and Chris Krogermeier for their support and guidance.

Deep appreciation to Chef Thomas Keller for his thoughtful foreword—and constant inspiration. And a special thanks to all the chefs who have shared their recipes with us—and *Men's Health* readers.

From Adina:
To my father, who took me to Reading Terminal Market when I was little and sent me to cooking school when I grew up. To my mother, who shared her love of chicken feet and other delicacies with me. And to my sister, who has grown from coconspirator in childhood taco concoctions to the woman I love to dine with most of all.

From Paul:
My heartfelt thanks to my mother, who taught me a love of cooking, my father, who taught me a love of eating, and the love of my life, who will always cook and eat with me.

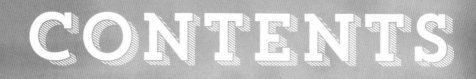

CONTENTS

1 WHAT'S COOKING? 1

Great meals don't happen by accident. They require
inspiration, planning, and good ingredients, plus the
tools and skills to prepare them right.

2 BREAKFAST 21

Wake up and smell the protein!

3 LUNCH 47

We've come a long way from the humble PB&J.

6 COOKING FOR A CROWD 125

Round up the crew. These big-batch meals are designed
to feed the masses.

7 EATING OUTSIDE

From grilling to barbecuing to camp cookery, here's how to make yourself the lord of the fires.

8 DATE NIGHT

As long as the food is good and you make the evening all about her, you'll earn four stars, chef.

9 CELEBRATION MEALS 237

Party smarter with holiday meals that won't wipe you out or weigh you down.

10 DRINKS 264

A guide to imbibing.

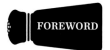

When man first discovered fire, he was quick to realize that the meats and vegetables he foraged in the wild tasted more appetizing with the application of heat. The high temperature lent a marked improvement in their flavor, texture and mouthfeel. Through trial and error, early man mastered the use of fire and utilized the craft of cooking to feed himself and others to have the energy to hunt and forage again and to thrive. In the modern world, we have transcended this natural instinct to prepare food solely for sustenance. We now cook for a myriad of reasons: to entertain, to relax, to bond, to impress, to fulfill our desire to nurture—even to seduce.

The dishes and recipes included in *Guy Gourmet,* the cookbook from *Men's Health* magazine, are a must for one's own survival today. They are important to master not only because they are healthful meals that taste wonderful, but because they will become a springboard for more complex cooking techniques. As with anything worthwhile, practice makes all the difference. It is only through the act of repetition that we develop muscle memory. Once our bodies become accustomed to the proper way of doing something, our brains are free to be inspired by everything else around us. We become adept at interpreting these recipes into something that is meaningful and personal to us, and in the process we evolve into better cooks ourselves.

Preparing good food begins with mastering simple skills that all chefs rely upon every day, skills like breaking down a chicken (page 171), grilling fish so it stays moist (page 183), knowing the tricks to cooking for more than four people (see Cooking for a Crowd, chapter 6), and even poaching an egg (page 24). If you want to enjoy Sirloin Steaks with Bacon–Blue Cheese Butter (page 137) the way The Meat Hook in Brooklyn does them, you need to start with a slab of sirloin and cut them yourself. To impress her with an affogato (page 233), it's all about the way to drizzle the hot espresso over the vanilla ice cream.

The resulting successes we encounter through practice and repetition give us the confidence and the courage to try new things. (Be sure to try Eric Ripert's delicious Grilled Tuna with Sauce Vierge, page 184.) Cooking is a life skill that will reap tremendous rewards—whether preparing us for crafting more intricate dishes or, more important, in learning how to cook healthier to achieve a balanced lifestyle. Raising our own awareness of what we put into our bodies ensures that the food we consume is nutritious and beneficial.

For these compelling reasons and perhaps a few of your own, it is time to browse through the index of these thoughtfully selected recipes, tie on an apron, and sharpen your knife. Enjoy the cooking process while forging ahead. Because, as our ancestors have certainly proven, trial and error can lead to many great accomplishments.

Thomas Keller
THE FRENCH LAUNDRY

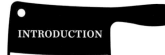

PASS THE NAPKINS

WE LOVE TO EAT. We love to cook. We love the way good food, prepared ourselves, makes us feel inside—whole, if not healthier. In the past 5 years, food and cooking have become increasingly important to the *Men's Health* brand—in our magazine, in our books and digital products, and in our 43 international editions.

Men's Health has always been a leader in reporting and writing about nutrition and the power of food to fuel and heal our bodies. But man does not live on steel-cut oatmeal and sockeye salmon alone. He needs . . . chili and steak, chicken soup and jambalaya. He must, on occasion, have barbecued ribs. And hot dogs, upgraded with gourmet toppings.

Yeah, even hot dogs. Because in our world, healthy eating means indulging in one of life's greatest joys—that is, lusciously decadent and satisfying food—some of the time, while eating lots of plants, fresh proteins, and other whole foods most of the time. It's about creating a healthy balance in an American diet that is heavily weighted toward the fast and processed.

So this cookbook, *Guy Gourmet,* is not a diet book despite the fact that it comes from Rodale, the world's leading seller of health books and publisher of *Men's Health, Women's Health,* and *Prevention* magazines. Its purpose is not to help you lose 30 pounds in 30 days. You won't find recipes substituting margarine for butter or nonfat cheese for the good stuff. In fact, you'll even bump into a few meals that might make a cardiologist wince even as he licks his lips and reaches for a fork. That said, if you take the recipes from this book and work them into your regular mealtime routine, you'll see benefits. You'll know exactly what ingredients you're putting into your body (you chopped them up!), you'll feast on delicious vegetables (cooked the way you like them), and, yes, we can almost guarantee that you will lose weight and build muscle by swapping your current meal plan for more *Guy Gourmet* fare. (Look for the recipes tagged with icons indicating extra health benefits!)

How can we be so sure about our grilled cheese and hardy side dishes? Well, consider this: If you cook more of your meals at home, you'll eat fewer meals outside your home, where a line cook hidden behind a wall is dishing up who-knows-what's-inside. Government studies have shown that when Americans eat a meal at a restaurant, they consume more calories and eat less nutritious food than they would if they prepared a meal and ate at home. Replace fast-food stops with home-cooked meals and you'll save hundreds of empty calories, fill up on more nutrients, and start trimming some inches off your waistline. Heck, cook at home and you can still have dessert!

Call it a tastier approach to losing weight and being healthier by eating better food. Delicious food. Remember, many of the recipes and tips inside this book come from the top chefs in the nation—cooks like Eric Ripert, Tyler Florence, Rick Bayless, Thomas Keller, John Besh, and Iron Chef Masaharu Morimoto. So, as a bonus, you'll be learning from the best of the best.

And once you start cooking more for yourself, other people reap the benefits, too. You'll be the customer who knows how to talk to his butcher. You'll be the man who melts a woman's heart with homemade pancakes on a Sunday. You'll be the guy who dishes out bowls of his famous chili at halftime, to rave reviews. And who doesn't want to be that guy?

—ADINA STEIMAN AND PAUL KITA

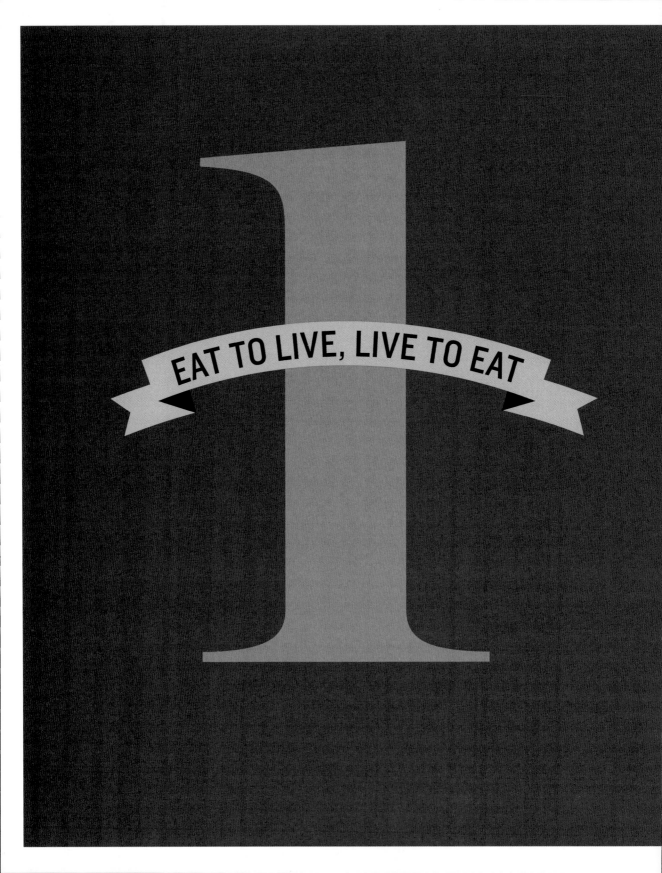

WHAT'S COOKING?

Great meals don't happen by accident. They require inspiration, accident. They require inspiration, planning, and good ingredients, plus the tools and skills to prepare them right.

Eating better starts long before you lift a fork. The first step is understanding what good food is and what healthier eating really means. After all, the advice seems to change with the weather, which results in a lot of confusion. Let's clear things up.

IF YOU WANT TO EAT HEALTHIER *(and lose some weight)*, EAT LESS.

You can eat really well and not have to worry about counting calories if you stick to a proper serving. Most of us don't understand portion control. We're eating double and even triple serving sizes, certainly at restaurants but even at home. Wait a couple of minutes before automatically reaching for seconds. The craving will likely pass.

NOT ALL CALORIES ARE CREATED EQUAL.

Your body's fuel comes from three sources: protein, carbohydrates, and fat. Your body metabolizes each of these macronutrients differently. For example, for every 100 carbohydrate calories you consume, your body expends only 5 to 10 in the process of digestion. This is officially called the thermic effect of food. By contrast, protein is the calorie-burn champ: For every 100 protein calories you consume, your body uses up 20 to 30 calories just to break that protein down. So, by eating protein instead of carbs, your body will end up with fewer calories to store after digestion is done. Fat is another story: Metabolizing fat requires even fewer calories than carbohydrates, about 3 for every 100 calories. But fat is more satiating than carbohydrates are. This nutrient stays in the gut longer, so it keeps you feeling full so you can say no to seconds. Protein keeps you full longer, too, and since it burns the most calories during digestion, it should figure into most of your meals.

As a general target, shoot for 20 to 40 grams of protein at each meal. Protein is a muscle builder. If you're looking to bulk up, your protein goal should be higher—about 1 gram of protein for each pound of target body weight you want to reach. It also matters what kind of protein you're eating. Many foods, including nuts and beans, can provide a good dose of protein. But the best sources are dairy products, eggs, meat, and fish. Animal protein is complete—it contains the right proportions of the essential amino acids your body can't synthesize on its own.

FAT IS NOT YOUR FOE.

It's unfortunate that dietary fat and the fat rolling over a fat man's belt are called the same thing. Many people still believe that eating fat will make you fat. It's a myth, caused by the demonizing of dietary fat by researchers who connected it to high cholesterol and heart disease. Unfortunately, the low-fat craze this thinking spawned substituted more sugar and refined grains for fats in our diets. Since 1971, intake of these unhealthy foods has expanded our daily calorie total by 168—and by extension, our waistlines.

Dietary fat is essential to good health. Omega-3 fats from oily fish are good for the heart and the brain. Monounsaturated fats, like those found in avocados and olive oil, will help improve your cholesterol profile and ease inflammation and arthritis symptoms. Even saturated fats, such as those found in steak, dark meat chicken, bacon, and butter, are important for good health. Research shows that saturated fat does not raise bad cholesterol levels. Plus, don't forget that fat makes foods taste great!

SUGAR IS DEADLY.

If you want to point a finger at the true type 2 diabetes culprit, it's sugar, sweet beverages like soda and juice, high-fructose corn syrup, white bread and other refined grains, and baked goods. Here's the problem with these foods:

Their sugars enter your bloodstream very rapidly. When you drink a can of soda, all of its sugar—all 12 to 20 teaspoons—goes directly into your blood, and those calories that you don't use immediately for energy will be stored as fat. This can lead to insulin resistance and diabetes, as the sugar overload overwhelms your body's ability to bring your blood sugar levels back to normal.

FIBER MAKES SUGARS SAFE.

Kidney beans contain sugar. But if you eat a soda's worth of sugar in kidney beans, it won't have the same dangerous effect as the liquid. That's because the sugar from kidney beans enters your blood slowly, thanks to the fiber content in those beans. Because it passes through your body undigested, fiber slows the absorption of sugar and other nutrients and makes you feel fuller longer, according to a study by researchers at the University of Minnesota. You don't need to eat bowls of beans and bran flakes every day to achieve this effect—just aim for 25 to 35 grams of fiber daily. Favor whole, unprocessed foods like most fruits and vegetables, legumes, and whole grains.

SALT ISN'T ALWAYS EVIL.

Actually, salt is essential to your health. Your body can't make it, and your cells need it to function. The sodium in salt is an electrolyte, a humble member of that hyped class of minerals that help maintain muscle function and hydration; that's why sports drinks contain sodium. You're constantly losing sodium through sweat and urine, and if you don't replenish that sodium and water, your blood pressure may drop far enough to make you dizzy and light-headed. If you have high blood pressure, you've probably been advised to cut back on salt. The mechanism seems clear: Sodium causes your blood to hold more water, so your heart has to pump harder, making your blood pressure rise. But what if you're a healthy guy? Tossing some salt into your pasta water isn't likely to send your blood pressure soaring. That's because 77 percent of the sodium in the average diet comes from processed and restaurant foods, according to the Centers for Disease Control and Prevention. (Just think about how thirsty you feel about an hour after a fast-food meal.) Only 12 percent of sodium is naturally occurring in foods, and just 5 percent comes from home cooking. Compliments to the chef.

GENTLEMEN, STOCK *your* PANTRY

Want to automatically eat healthier? Stock up on the healthiest foods. From hunting down the right ingredients to storing them skillfully, the strategies you use to bring food into your kitchen can make all the difference.

RULE 1
MASTER YOUR IMPULSES

Easy-grab items at the market tend to be built from bottom-of-the-barrel ingredients—sugar, starch, and cheap fats. Use these strategies to resist their siren song.

GRAB A CART A study in the *Journal of Marketing Research* shows that shopping with a basket instead of a cart makes you nearly seven times more likely to purchase vice foods like candy and chocolate. The researchers say that curling your arm inward to carry a basket increases your desire to embrace instant rewards—like sweet foods. With a cart, you tend to extend your arms—a motion associated with avoiding negative outcomes. That makes you more likely to shop smart.

AVOID THE LINES The longer you're exposed to tempting salty and chocolaty snacks at the checkout, the more likely you are to succumb to them, say University of Arizona researchers. Avoid the wait by shopping during off-peak times, such as the middle of the week or late at night.

LEAVE THE KIDS AT HOME "Children shouldn't have a vote in supermarket decisions," says Greg Critser, author of *Fat Land: How Americans Became the Fattest People in the World.* That includes your inner child. About 80 percent of parents report that they'll probably buy snacks or frozen desserts if their kids ask for them at the grocery store, according to a 2011 Mintel report.

RULE 2
IGNORE THE PACKAGING BILLBOARDS

Time for a turnaround. "The front of a food package is real estate owned by the manufacturer, whose goal is to sell you something," says *Men's Health* weight-loss advisor David Katz, M.D., M.P.H. Flip the package over to find the information you need on the one part that's well regulated by the FDA: the Nutrition Facts label.

RULE 3
WORK THE PERIMETER

The inner aisles of the store are where you'll find the unhealthiest of foods. Stick to the outskirts for the bulk of your ingredients. That's where the fresh stuff is found—meats and seafood, fruits and vegetables. Hang out there more.

HOW TO PICK THE PERFECT PRODUCE

The best isn't always the prettiest. Imperfections can be attractive, hinting at surprising sweetness and depth of character.

We're talking about food, by the way. Too many supermarkets sell produce bred not for taste, but to withstand shipping—it's well-shaped, but not flavorful. You want your fruit to be naturally voluptuous; the farmer's daughter, not the plasticized porn star.

EMPLOY YOUR SENSES.

LOOK:

Prime fruits and vegetables are often irregularly shaped and blemished.

TOUCH:

Heavy, sturdy fruits and vegetables with taut skin are freshest.

SMELL:

Many fruits can be sniffed for ripeness.

AND SHOP SEASONALLY:

The foods are tastier and cheaper.

ORGANIZE YOUR FRIDGE

One of the easiest ways to upgrade your diet is to rearrange your refrigerator. How you position your groceries may shape the way you eat.

SHELVE STRATEGICALLY

Fill your eye-level shelf (or top shelf) with fruits, vegetables, and other nutritious snacks. You're 2.7 times more likely to eat healthy food if it's in your line of sight, a Cornell University study says. "That's also why manufacturers pay a premium to have their products at eye level in stores," says Kit Yarrow, Ph.D., a professor of psychology and marketing at Golden Gate University.

PACK SMART

A variety of small leftover containers tempts you to eat more than you had planned, says Brian Wansink, Ph.D., author of *Mindless Eating: Why We Eat More Than We Think.* Instead, combine leftover entrées and sides so that each container has one meal's worth.

SHOP MORE, BUY LESS

Instead of laying in supplies for the week, hit the supermarket more often and buy only for the next few meals. An overload of choices at home may deplete your willpower, a 2008 *Journal of Consumer Psychology* study found. "And people tend to reduce consumption when resources are scarce," Yarrow says.

HIDE THE JUNK

All stocked up on snacks? Now make sure you eat the good ones. In a 2009 Danish study, one in four participants who chose a healthy snack over an unhealthy one later reached for the junk anyway. So place the healthy stuff front and center, and stash small guilty pleasures out of sight.

SMARTER STORAGE

Food lasts longer when it's stored properly. Follow these tips from Nils Noren, vice president of culinary and pastry arts at the French Culinary Institute.

1 Set your fridge temp at just above freezing, around 34°F. That's cold enough to slow the growth of bacteria without freezing the food.

2 Put items with short shelf lives in the back. Milk, meat, fish, and eggs last longer in the back because that's where refrigerators are coldest—and that way they'll also be protected from a blast of warm air every time you open the door, says Noren.

3 Stash raw proteins on the lowest shelf so no meat juices can drip onto other shelves and season your food with pathogens, says Noren. And wipe down your fridge at least once a week with a disinfecting wipe or a clean cloth dipped in a solution of soap, water, and a little bleach.

HARDWARE *and* BUILDING SUPPLIES

You wouldn't tune up a motorcycle or attempt to hang a door without the right tools. That would only result in frustration and a shoddy job. Same goes for cooking. To make incredible meals, you need good gear. You can go nuts with kitchen gadgets, as anyone who has ever received a Williams-Sonoma catalog can attest. But just as you don't need a Powermatic Jet 2000 table saw with Rout-R-Lift to cut a few 2 x 4s, you can get by nicely in the kitchen with a handful of basic tools. Here is a common inventory of a cooking man's kitchen workshop.

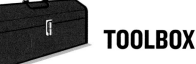

THE KITCHEN TOOLBOX

SHOPSPEAK	CHEFSPEAK	SHOPSPEAK	CHEFSPEAK
Saw	**Chef's knife**	Pliers	**Tongs**
T-square	**Measuring spoons/cups**	File	**Grater**
Hammer	**Mallet**	Screen	**Colander**
X-Acto knife	**Paring knife**	Bucket	**Mixing bowl**
Plane	**Potato peeler**	Multitool	**Can opener**
Workbench	**Cutting board**	Blowtorch	**Caramelizing torch**
Portable drill	**Hand beater**	Circular saw	**Food processor**
Drill press	**Mixer**		

the ESSENTIALS

You don't have to purchase a full toolbox of kitchen gadgets to start making great meals. Add to your arsenal as you go. But here are the key essentials to start off right and why you need them.

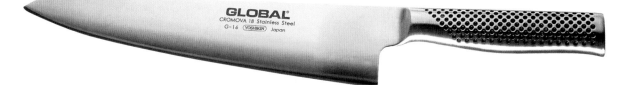

1 AN 8" OR 10" CHEF'S KNIFE

It's the hands-down most important tool a cook needs in his kitchen. Work with a crappy knife and you'll cook crappy food or—worse yet—dice off a digit. A trusty chef's knife will chop, mince, carve, fillet, slice, and dice nearly any ingredient. Why the option of 8 or 10 inches? The longer the knife, the sturdier it is and the more powerful its hacking ability, but the heavier its weight. When you buy a knife, always ask to hold it before breaking out your cash. If it feels like an extension of your arm, it's a good fit. Too heavy? Opt for a smaller blade length.

To pick a knife that's right for you, see "Choose Your Weapon," page 13.

the **ESSENTIALS**

2 A PARING KNIFE

A chef's knife is your most trusted kitchen sidekick, but sometimes it's too powerful for its own good. To tackle more tedious kitchen tasks (coring bell peppers, de-stemming tomatoes, deveining shrimp), pick up this more compact blade, which is usually $2\frac{1}{2}$ to 4 inches long.

3 A BREAD KNIFE

The serrated edge of this blade won't massacre crusty loaves of fresh bread like even the best chef's knives tend to do. No need to splurge for anything fancy here. A bread knife is a bread knife.

5 A CAST-IRON SKILLET

When you can't grill outside, use this sturdy standby to help you sear burgers and steaks to juicy perfection. Remember to never clean cast iron with soap and water, because you'll ruin the "seasoning" seal on the pan. Wipe it clean with paper towels or, for caked-on gunk, pour some kosher salt onto the surface and scrub. Reseason afterwards with a bit of oil.

4 TWO SIZES OF NONSTICK SAUTÉ PANS

Pick up a large and a small version—you'll be doing the majority of your stovetop cooking on these. The two sizes can help you tag-team a dinner of seared salmon and a vegetable side. Bonus: You can use both pans simultaneously to create a panini press. Just place the sandwich you want pressed on the bottom pan, and then weigh down the pan on top of the sandwich with heavy books or cans. Infomercial gadgets be damned.

6 TWO SIZES OF STAINLESS STEEL MIXING BOWLS

Whether you're making a big batch of dip for game day, tossing salad greens with homemade dressing, or mixing the ingredients of a BBQ ribs rub, you'll need a container for the task at hand. These bowls can take a beating, come in handy for a variety of kitchen jobs, and are simple to clean.

7 A WOODEN SPOON

Metal can scratch your nonstick sauté pans and cast iron skillet. An inexpensive wooden spoon will help you sauté without causing damage to your valuable kitchen hardware.

9 A MEAT THERMOMETER

A foodborne illness is a lousy excuse for declining dessert. Avoid that experience by purchasing this simple piece of kitchen hardware. Depend on it and you'll cook perfect protein, every time. (For a temperature guide for meats, turn to page 18.)

10 TONGS

For flipping steaks, burgers, vegetables, and—in case of emergencies—opening beer bottles.

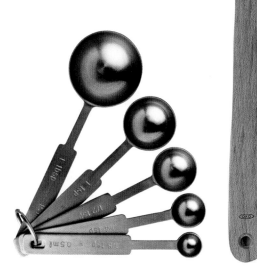

8 MEASURING SPOONS/CUPS

After you cook for a while, you'll gain an ability to judge a recipe's components by taste and be able to estimate quantities. Until then, leave the precision to these tools.

11 A SPATULA

You'll be using yours to stir sauces, mix stir-fry, scramble eggs, and more. Avoid spatulas with wooden handles, which tend to rot after repeated exposure to water.

the ESSENTIALS

12 A FOOD PROCESSOR

For heavy-duty salsa making, pesto pureeing, hummus whirring, and spice pulverization, you're going to need blades that can work quickly.

13 A SLOW COOKER

It's extremely versatile and easy to use: Just prep the ingredients the night before, put them into the pot before you leave for work in the morning, and when you come home, you have dinner. And since the pot is heavy-bottomed, the heat is dispersed evenly, so you have less chance of burning your food.

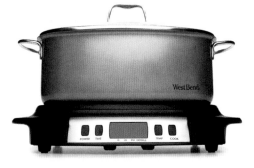

14 A CUTTING BOARD

Go with wood. Although plastic is nonporous, you're likely to put deeper knife marks into it, making it hard to clean. Also, wood won't dull your knives as quickly, and it draws bacteria below the surface—and therefore away from your food. In fact, a study by researchers at the University of California, Davis, Food Safety Laboratory found that used, scarred wooden cutting boards had almost the same amount of bacteria on their surfaces as new wooden ones.

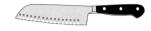

THE KNIFE YOU DON'T NEED

Despite what Rachael Ray says, skip the Japanese-style santoku blade. These knives are often too short and light to cut as deftly as a 10" chef's knife. "If pressed, I might use it for light tasks, like chopping mushrooms or dicing celery," says Norman Weinstein, author of *Mastering Knife Skills*.

CHOOSE YOUR WEAPON

RUN THIS DIAGNOSTIC TO DISCOVER THE BEST CHEF'S KNIFE FOR YOU

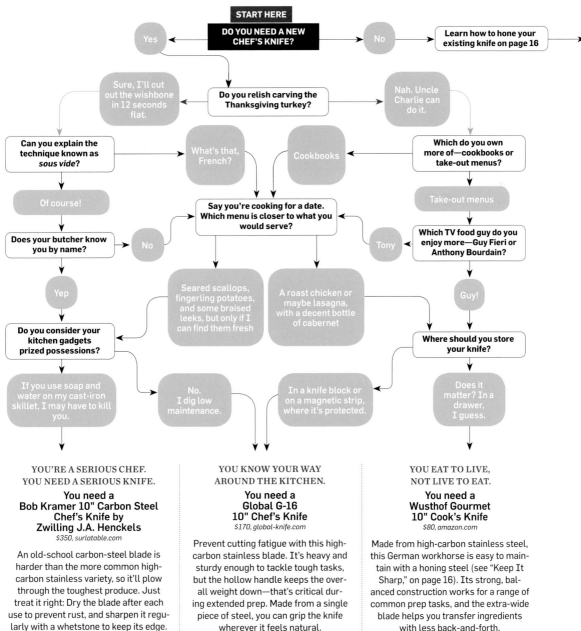

START HERE

DO YOU NEED A NEW CHEF'S KNIFE?

Yes ← → No → **Learn how to hone your existing knife on page 16**

Do you relish carving the Thanksgiving turkey?

Sure, I'll cut out the wishbone in 12 seconds flat.

Nah. Uncle Charlie can do it.

Can you explain the technique known as *sous vide*?

What's that, French?

Cookbooks

Which do you own more of—cookbooks or take-out menus?

Of course!

Say you're cooking for a date. Which menu is closer to what you would serve?

Take-out menus

Does your butcher know you by name?

No

Which TV food guy do you enjoy more—Guy Fieri or Anthony Bourdain?

Yep

Tony

Seared scallops, fingerling potatoes, and some braised leeks, but only if I can find them fresh

A roast chicken or maybe lasagna, with a decent bottle of cabernet

Guy!

Do you consider your kitchen gadgets prized possessions?

Where should you store your knife?

If you use soap and water on my cast-iron skillet, I may have to kill you.

No. I dig low maintenance.

In a knife block or on a magnetic strip, where it's protected.

Does it matter? In a drawer, I guess.

YOU'RE A SERIOUS CHEF. YOU NEED A SERIOUS KNIFE.

You need a Bob Kramer 10" Carbon Steel Chef's Knife by Zwilling J.A. Henckels
$350, surlatable.com

An old-school carbon-steel blade is harder than the more common high-carbon stainless variety, so it'll plow through the toughest produce. Just treat it right: Dry the blade after each use to prevent rust, and sharpen it regularly with a whetstone to keep its edge.

YOU KNOW YOUR WAY AROUND THE KITCHEN.

You need a Global G-16 10" Chef's Knife
$170, global-knife.com

Prevent cutting fatigue with this high-carbon stainless blade. It's heavy and sturdy enough to tackle tough tasks, but the hollow handle keeps the over-all weight down—that's critical during extended prep. Made from a single piece of steel, you can grip the knife wherever it feels natural.

YOU EAT TO LIVE, NOT LIVE TO EAT.

You need a Wusthof Gourmet 10" Cook's Knife
$80, amazon.com

Made from high-carbon stainless steel, this German workhorse is easy to maintain with a honing steel (see "Keep It Sharp," on page 16). Its strong, balanced construction works for a range of common prep tasks, and the extra-wide blade helps you transfer ingredients with less back-and-forth.

HOW
to COOK

Most men do just fine in life making things up as they go along. While that may work in business, it won't cut it when it comes to cooking. A man needs instructions. This book delivers easy-to-follow recipes, plus the how-to for basic techniques that'll help you turn a list of ingredients and cook times into delicious and impressive meals.

MASTER THE KEY SKILLS

Chefs can make cooking look complicated, but most recipes come down to these five basic techniques. Learn more about them here, use them often, and they'll become second nature.

ROASTING

Roasting employs the dry, indirect heat of the oven to add a tasty crust to meat or to brown a pan of vegetables. It's also a great way to intensify the natural sweetness of fruits and vegetables.

KEY TO SUCCESS: To ensure great browning, don't overcrowd the roasting pan and make sure your ingredients are coated with a light film of oil.

BROILING/ GRILLING

Man's first cooking technique may also be his most flavorful. Whether you heat from the top, using the broiler, or from underneath, on the grill, the food acquires a tasty crust. This works well with meats, of course, but also with fish, vegetables, and pizza.

KEY TO SUCCESS: Watch your food like a hawk. Food under the broiler or on the grill can go from juicy to scorched in an instant.

BRAISING

Braising is the technique responsible for the most tender meats and the most complex flavors. To begin, brown the meat on the stovetop. Then turn down the heat and cook the ingredients in a small amount of liquid until very tender. Once everything's in the pan, braising requires little or no effort from you.

KEY TO SUCCESS: To ensure a tender braise, make sure the liquid is gently simmering, rather than boiling.

BOILING

Put food in water. Boil until done. You, too, can employ this technique for a healthy vegetable soup, perfectly cooked pasta, and more.

KEY TO SUCCESS: To bring water to a boil fast, don't forget to cover the pot. And always season the water with salt (plenty of salt, for pasta)— you'll infuse flavor right into the food.

SAUTÉING

Sautéing simply means cooking in a pan with butter or oil over fairly high heat, developing gently browned edges and keeping the insides juicy.

KEY TO SUCCESS: Unless you're cooking garlic, which burns easily, always start with a hot pan, add oil or butter, let it heat briefly, and then add the food. If the food doesn't sizzle, your pan's not hot enough.

KNOW YOUR KNIFE

Cutting up your ingredients might seem like a tedious exercise—something to plod through before the real cooking begins. But learning how to wield your knife precisely doesn't just make you look impressive—it also helps your food cook evenly. A few general principles before you start:

RULE 1
SOURCE THE BEST TOOLS.

Invest in a sturdy cutting board and a good-quality chef's knife (see page 13 to find the best one for you), and every slice will be easier.

RULE 2
DON'T BLEED.

Make sure your knife is sharp—dull knives are more likely to slip and cause injury. And always tuck your fingertips under as you grip the ingredient you're cutting.

RULE 3
USE THE RIGHT PART OF THE BLADE.

The tip of your chef's knife is perfect for closely spaced precision cuts. The middle of your knife works best for chopping and overall slicing. And the heavy base of your knife is great for muscling through tough root vegetables.

KEEP IT SHARP

Even the best knives become dull with use. The good news: You can keep a chef's knife factory-sharp with a honing steel. Remember, sharpening will restore a knife's edge; honing maintains it. If your blade has already lost its edge, have a professional bring it back to life. Otherwise, hone it by following these three steps from knife expert Norman Weinstein.

1 Select a medium-grit, oval-shaped honing steel that's 2" longer than your knife. (An oval shape allows for more surface contact with the knife than a round steel does.) Buy one from the German company Dick (dick.de).

2 Grasp the steel's handle and place the tip on your counter or cutting board. Hold the knife against the steel at a 20-degree angle.

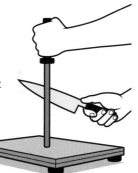

3 Place the knife's heel near the top of the steel. Using moderate pressure, pull the knife back and down from heel to tip, from the top of the steel to the bottom. Remember not to turn your wrist during the motion—that false move will change the angle. Four or five strokes on each side will revive your blade.

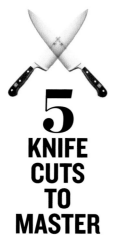

5 KNIFE CUTS TO MASTER

SLICING PEPPERS

1 Cut off the very top and bottom of the pepper. Then cut it in half vertically.

2 Lay each half on a cutting board, skin side down, and slide your knife across the curved inner surface, removing the ribs and their seeds. Follow the curve of the flesh to avoid cutting off more than is necessary.

3 While holding a pepper half on the cutting board, rock your chef's knife back and forth, moving down the length of the pepper to cut slices to your desired width.

DICING CARROTS

1 Peel the carrot and then cut a 3" log from the fatter end.

2 Trim off four sides to shape the piece into a rectangular block.

3 Place the piece on one of its sides and cut ¼"-wide slices lengthwise, keeping your fingers in a clawlike grasp (fingernails tucked in) on the carrot.

4 Stack those slabs and cut ¼"-wide strips lengthwise. Then cut crosswise to form ¼" cubes. (Note: Feel free to adjust the size of the dice to suit the recipe.)

CHOPPING ONIONS

1 Halve the onion from top to bottom, but don't trim off the root end.

2 Peel one onion half and place the flat side on a cutting board.

3 Use the blade to cut almost to the stem end, but not through, in ½" increments along the onion.

4 Use the blade to slice down perpendicular to those horizontal cuts you just made, yielding neat ½" cubes.

MINCING GARLIC

1 Separate a head of garlic into cloves.

2 Place one clove of unpeeled garlic on your work surface and position the blade of a chef's knife flat on top of the garlic.

3 Use the heel of your hand to hit the blade lightly, smashing the clove.

4 Remove the loosened peel and rock the knife back and forth over the flattened garlic, chopping until the garlic is reduced to small bits.

CHOPPING HERBS

1 Strip the leaves of the herbs from their stems and place them on a cutting board.

2 Mount the leaves into a pile and begin rocking the blade of your chef's knife back and forth over the herbs, using the palm of your other hand to help the knife rock on its curve.

3 Continue rocking the blade over the herbs until they reach the desired size.

MASTER THE PROTEINS

Sure, after you've cooked countless cuts of meat, fowl, and fish, you might begin to develop a near-magical ability to gauge doneness by touch or sight alone. But for most of us mere mortals, the best way to cook perfectly done protein every time is to deploy a trusty instant-read thermometer—and know the ideal temperature target for each type of protein. A few guidelines before you start:

RULE 1
Be sure to turn on the thermometer and allow it to calibrate before inserting the probe into the meat.

RULE 2
In general, aim for the center of the cut of meat, since that's where it's least cooked.

RULE 3
With larger cuts of meat, the internal temperature will continue to rise after you finish cooking. Pull larger cuts off when they're a few degrees shy of their target temperature to compensate for this.

CHICKEN
whole or pieces

COOK IT
6 to 8 minutes each side

IT'S DONE
165°F

RESTING TIME
5 minutes for pieces,
10 minutes for whole

BEEF
roasts; thick bone-in steaks (porterhouse, T-bone); thin boneless steaks (flank, skirt)

COOK IT
10 to 12 minutes each side for thick, 4 to 6 minutes each side for thin

IT'S DONE
145°F (medium-rare)

RESTING TIME
15 minutes for roasts,
5 minutes for steaks

FISH FILLETS
such as salmon

COOK IT
2 minutes flesh side down, then 6 to 8 minutes skin side down

IT'S DONE
Skip the thermometer.
Look for opaque, defined stripes along the top and sides.

RESTING TIME
In general, by the time the fish hits your plate, it's rested enough.

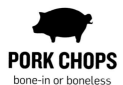

PORK CHOPS
bone-in or boneless

COOK IT
5 to 7 minutes each side for
boneless, 5 to 10 minutes for
bone-in

IT'S DONE
145°F (medium)

RESTING TIME
5 minutes for thin chops,
15 minutes for thick ones

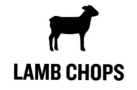

LAMB CHOPS

COOK IT
3 to 4 minutes on each side

IT'S DONE
140–145°F (medium-rare)

RESTING TIME
5 minutes for thin chops,
15 minutes for thick ones

HOW TO USE THIS BOOK

So now you have the nutritional know-how, the supermarket smarts, the gear, and the skills you need to start cooking. To help you find the recipes you need, fast, we've included symbols that'll tip you off to the unique benefits of certain meals. Here's a key to guide you.

MUSCLE BUILDER

These meals contain high amounts of protein per serving. Consider them ammo for your guns.

TIME SAVER

Turn to these recipes when you're looking for a quick meal. Fast-food joints, beware.

HEART HELPER

Eat these meals and your heart will thank you for the whole grains, monounsaturated fats, and/or omega-3 fatty acids.

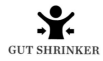

GUT SHRINKER

All the flavor for fewer calories—these dishes will help you stay lean or lose the weight you want.

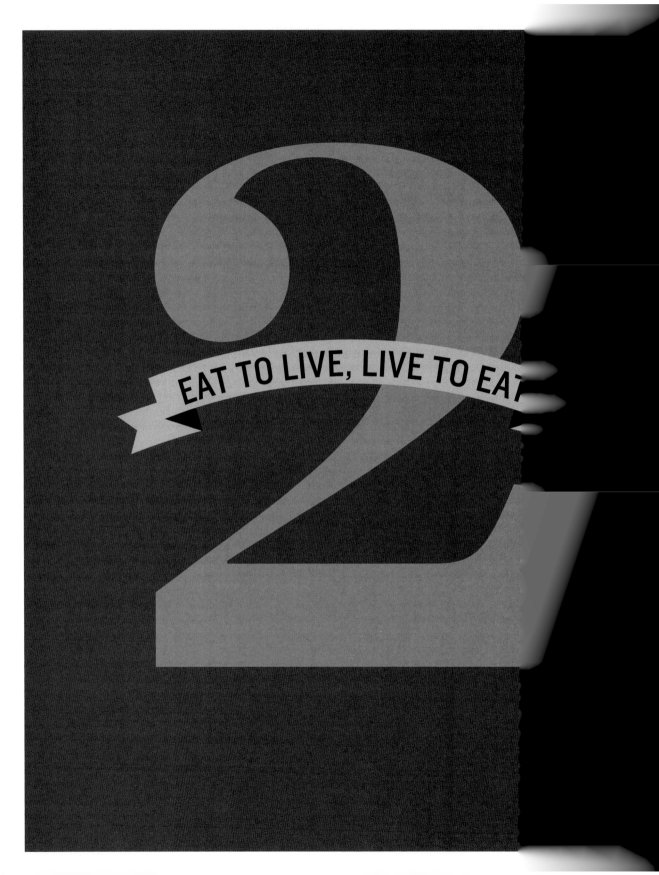

2

EAT TO LIVE, LIVE TO EAT

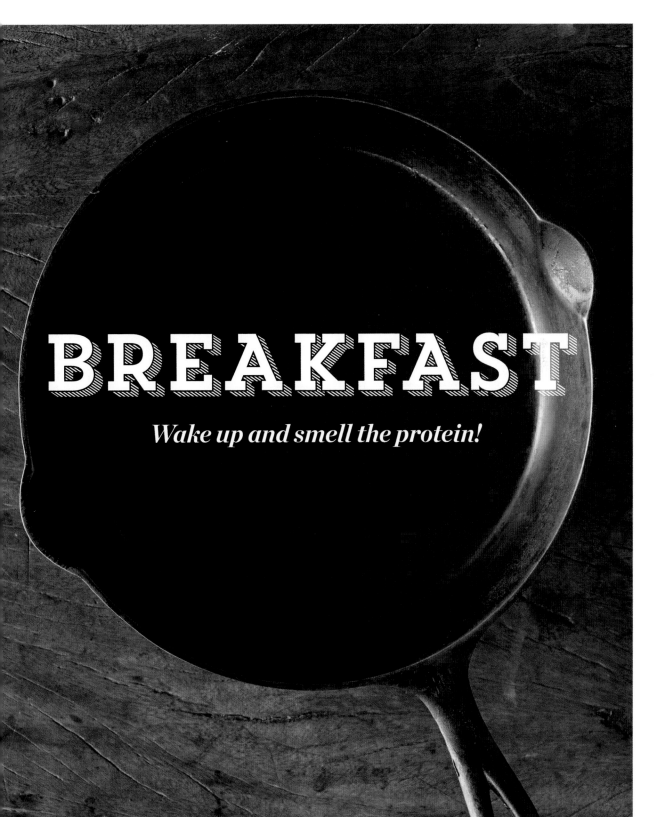

BREAKFAST

Wake up and smell the protein!

p. 22 · GUY MH GOURMET · c. 02

THE RULES *of* BREAKFAST

Those cereal commercials you used to watch during Saturday morning cartoons were only half right. Yes, you should start your day off with a well-balanced meal. Studies show that eating a solid breakfast will reduce the number of calories you eat over the course of the day, stave off excess snacking, and generally make you a healthier guy. Where the ad execs screwed things up? There are far better strategies to start off your day nutritionally than a bowlful of mini sugar-bombs. Read up, chow down.

RULE Nº.

1

WELL, EAT IT

WE KNOW. You're busy. Maybe you have time for a protein bar on the way out the door. But, look, if you want a lean, muscular body, you can't skip breakfast. Eating in the morning makes you less likely to overeat during the day because your blood sugar will remain steady—as long as you don't overdose on carbohydrates (more on this later). People who eat regularly report less stress, better focus, and fewer injuries and accidents at work, according to a British study published in the journal *Nutrients*. Think about it: You've fasted all night long—your brain needs fresh fuel to comprehend all those spreadsheets and red-flagged e-mails your boss sends.

RULE N<u>o.</u> 2 | PACK IN PROTEIN

SORRY, BUDDY, a granola bar just won't cut it. You need to eat protein, and plenty of it. That's because starting your day with plenty of protein triggers protein synthesis, a process that helps maintain and grow your muscles before you even lift the bar off the squat rack. This muscle-growing fuel raises the levels of peptides—synthesized amino acids—in your stomach. These aminos can help you feel fuller, longer throughout the day. We say aim for 20 to 40 grams of protein per breakfast.

And don't forget to pair your protein with some fat. That's because, along with protein, it slows the absorption of carbohydrates into your bloodstream, providing you with a steady supply of energy—instead of a quick sugar rush (often followed by a sugar crash). And by keeping you full longer, this protein/fat combo can also help shrink your midsection.

RULE N<u>o.</u> 3 | FILL UP ON FIBER

A GOOD BREAKFAST stays with you—all the way through to lunch. But that doesn't mean that you need to sit down to a massive lumberjack-style meal to stave off 11 a.m. hunger pangs. Just don't forget the fiber. Fiber slows the absorption of nutrients and makes you feel fuller longer. To reap the satiating benefits of fiber, aim for 25 to 35 grams daily, and avoid refined, low-fiber carbohydrates. Try adding fiber-rich vegetables to your omelets, kale to your smoothies, and chia seeds and fresh berries to your morning oatmeal.

RULE N<u>o.</u> 4 | PLAN AHEAD

THE BEAUTY OF breakfast is that you can make it in big batches—and then eat well all week long. In the recipes that follow, you can always double up a recipe, such as our awesome protein-loaded oatmeal (page 30), and stash it in the fridge to reheat all week. Or, whip up a bunch of almond waffles (page 31), freeze the extras, and then pop them in a toaster for when you only have a few moments to eat. If you cook ahead of time, you're more likely to eat the food you cook. And if you eat the food you cook, you're more likely to drive right past the fast-food drive-thru on the way to work.

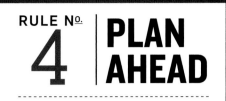

The Recipes

GREEN EGGS *and* HAM

Call it a Seussian approach to breakfast (or even dinner).
This ham-and-egg breakfast sandwich carries a punch of garlicky pesto
and a slight smokiness from roasted red peppers. To make only one
serving, just poach the desired number of eggs in the water and vinegar
bath, quartering the rest of the recipe.

1	tablespoon distilled white vinegar
8	eggs
2	tablespoons prepared pesto
2	tablespoons plain Greek yogurt
4	whole wheat English muffins, split
4–8	slices ham, prosciutto, or cooked Canadian bacon
¼	cup sliced jarred roasted red peppers
	Salt and ground black pepper

1. Bring 3" of water to a boil in a large skillet or wide saucepan. Reduce to a bare simmer and add the vinegar. Working in two batches, poach the eggs (see "The Laws of Poaching," below) until the whites are just firm, 3 to 5 minutes. Using a slotted spoon, remove the eggs to a plate.

2. In a small bowl, mix together the pesto and yogurt until they're smooth and combined. Toast the split English muffins until golden.

3. Dividing evenly, top 4 of the muffin halves with the ham, roasted peppers, and eggs. Season with salt and black pepper to taste and add the pesto mixture. Top the eggs with the remaining muffin halves.

MAKES 4 SERVINGS · PER SERVING **363** CALORIES // **17 G** FAT // **1,056 MG** SODIUM // **31 G** CARBOHYDRATES // **5 G** DIETARY FIBER // **24 G** PROTEIN

○ THE LAWS OF POACHING

There's no need to be intimidated by poaching eggs. It's an easy and essential breakfast (or brunch) skill that everyone should master.

1 Don't crack eggs directly into the water—you might break the yolks. Carefully crack one egg into a small bowl before adding it to the water (see Step 2); then repeat with the next egg.

2 Boiling makes eggs tough. Instead, bring water to a gentle simmer in a large skillet. Then add a spoonful of white vinegar—it helps the egg hold together. Move the bowl with the egg close to the water as you slip the egg in.

3 Cook the eggs until the whites are just firm, 3 to 5 minutes depending on the eggs' size. Use a slotted spoon to remove each egg carefully.

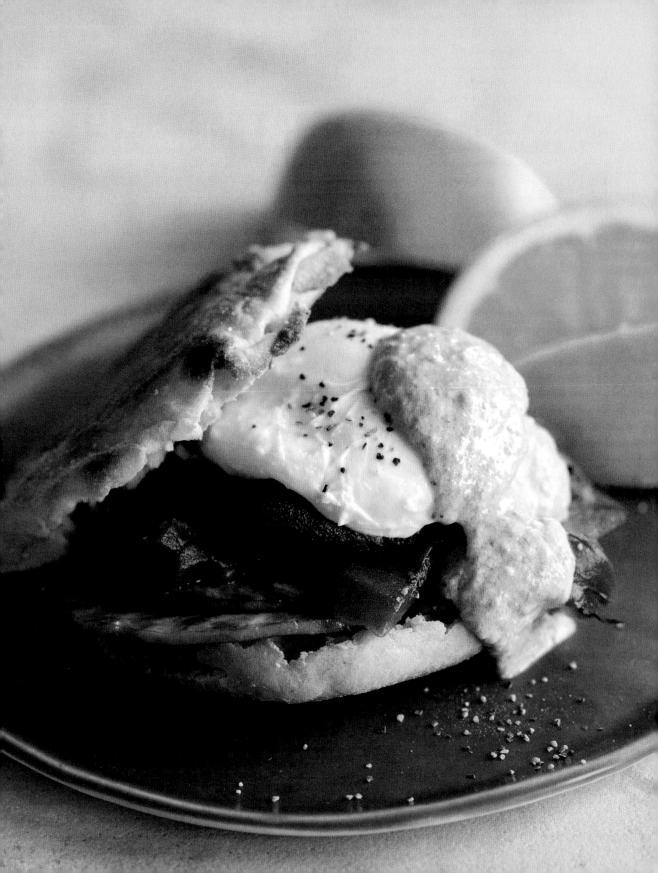

MAKE PERFECT OMELETS

Master the basics of the omelet and you can customize countless breakfasts. Learn how to cook the eggs just right and flip the omelet with the savvy of a diner line cook.

THE HEAT

Lightly coat a medium nonstick skillet with cooking spray. Turn the burner under the pan to medium-high, hot enough to cause discomfort when your hand's an inch above it.

THE SCRAMBLE

Whisk 2 eggs with 2 tablespoons of water and add a shake or two of salt. The salt breaks down the egg whites for an even smoother consistency. The water gives the eggs a fluffy texture. Stay away from milk. It can make the eggs heavy.

THE POUR

If you're cooking more than one omelet, mix the eggs all at once and use a soup ladle to pour the eggs.

THE SIMMER

Push cooked egg from the edges of the pan toward the center with your spatula, and tilt the pan so raw egg runs to the exposed metal. Then, when no more egg runs but the top of the omelet is still very moist, turn the handle toward you and sprinkle filling across the near half of the omelet, from 3 to 9 o'clock.

AND NOW . . . THE FLIP

Give the handle a jerk toward you. This will send the eggs up the far side of the pan. Push the handle back to its starting position as the omelet is halfway up over the lip of the pan. Your creation should fold in half, pretty as a picture. If at first you don't succeed, flip and flip again.

THE FILLING

Dice vegetables and meats into very small pieces—large chunks will cause the egg to tear when you flip it. Try…

**Roasted red peppers
(about ¼ cup)**

+

**Chopped grilled
asparagus (about ½ cup)**

PER SERVING: 166 CALORIES,
10 G FAT, 171 MG SODIUM, 6 G
CARBOHYDRATES, 1 G DIETARY
FIBER, 14 G PROTEIN

**Crumbled cooked
sausage (¼ cup)**

+

Chopped red bell pepper

+

Chopped onion (¼ cup)

PER SERVING: 253 CALORIES,
18 G FAT, 510 MG SODIUM, 4 G
CARBOHYDRATES, 0 G DIETARY
FIBER, 18 G PROTEIN

Smoked salmon (1 ounce)

+

**Chopped red onion
(2 tablespoons)**

+

Capers

+

**Chopped dill
(1 teaspoon each)**

PER SERVING: 195 CALORIES,
12 G FAT, 383 MG SODIUM, 3 G
CARBOHYDRATES, 0 G DIETARY
FIBER, 20 G PROTEIN

**Goat cheese
(2 tablespoons)**

+

**A mix of chopped
parsley and chives
(2 tablespoons)**

PER SERVING: 145 CALORIES,
10 G FAT, 143 MG SODIUM, 1 G
CARBOHYDRATES, 0 G DIETARY
FIBER, 13 G PROTEIN

Bacon (1 slice)

+

**Shredded cheddar
cheese (2 tablespoons)**

+

**A few dashes of your
favorite hot sauce**

PER SERVING: 240 CALORIES,
18 G FAT, 425 MG SODIUM, 1 G
CARBOHYDRATES, 0 G DIETARY
FIBER, 19 G PROTEIN

**Chopped sautéed
mushrooms (¼ cup)**

+

**A spoonful of
sour cream**

+

**Chopped parsley
(2 tablespoons)**

PER SERVING: 245 CALORIES,
20 G FAT, 478 MG SODIUM, 4 G
CARBOHYDRATES, 1 G DIETARY
FIBER, 15 G PROTEIN

THE ULTIMATE HANGOVER BREAKFAST

Rough night? Wake up with a breakfast of ham with red-eye gravy dish, which incorporates coffee into a bold-tasting gravy that goes great with thick-cut ham. And to drink? More coffee couldn't hurt.

Fry 2 thick slices of center-cut ham (about 6 ounces each) in a skillet with 2 tablespoons oil until lightly browned; remove them to a plate. Add fresh-brewed coffee to the pan (about the same amount as there is fat). Simmer, scraping up any browned bits, until the gravy thickens, 5 to 10 minutes. Pour the gravy over the ham. Serve with fried eggs and biscuits or whole wheat toast.

MAKES 2 SERVINGS

PER SERVING:
(HAM AND GRAVY ONLY)
469 CALORIES, 36 G FAT,
2,358 MG SODIUM, 0 G CARBOHY-
DRATES, 0 G DIETARY FIBER,
34 G PROTEIN

PUMPKIN PANCAKES

Your secret ingredient to better pancakes: canned pumpkin. It adds just
enough sweetness so you don't have to clobber your short stacks
with calorie-laden syrup. Canned or fresh, pumpkin is loaded with fiber,
beta-carotene, and incredible flavor. Use it to make these awesome
seasonal pancakes, courtesy of Jodi Hortze, owner of the Griddle Cafe
in Los Angeles. To boost your protein, pair the pancakes with a couple of
slices of crispy bacon or seared Canadian bacon.

2   cups dry pancake mix
     (your favorite)

3   tablespoons dark brown
     sugar

2½   teaspoons pumpkin pie
     spice

1½   cups milk

1   cup canned unsweetened
     pumpkin puree (not pie
     filling)

1   egg, beaten

1   teaspoon vanilla extract

1   tablespoon vegetable oil,
     plus more for the griddle

     Pure maple syrup

1. In a large bowl, combine the pancake mix, brown sugar, and
pumpkin pie spice. In another large bowl, mix together the milk,
pumpkin, egg, vanilla extract, and oil. Add the pumpkin mixture to the
dry ingredients and stir to combine.

2. Heat a lightly oiled griddle or large skillet over medium-high heat.
Pour the batter onto the griddle, using about ¼ cup for each pancake.
Cook the pancakes until bubbles form in the batter and the edges
begin to brown. Then flip them and cook until the other sides are
lightly browned.

3. Serve the pancakes drizzled with maple syrup.

MAKES 20 PANCAKES · PER SERVING/4 PANCAKES **404** CALORIES //
9 G FAT // **683 MG** SODIUM // **72 G** CARBOHYDRATES // **3 G** DIETARY FIBER // **10 G** PROTEIN

○ COOK PERFECT BACON

The secret to perfectly cooked bacon: Skip the pan or the skillet. Bacon's tendency to
scrunch up makes for uneven cooking. Instead, place no more than a half pound of bacon on an
18" x 12" rimmed baking sheet and roast in a 375°F oven for 12 to 15 minutes, for that perfectly
crisp (but not too crisp) texture.

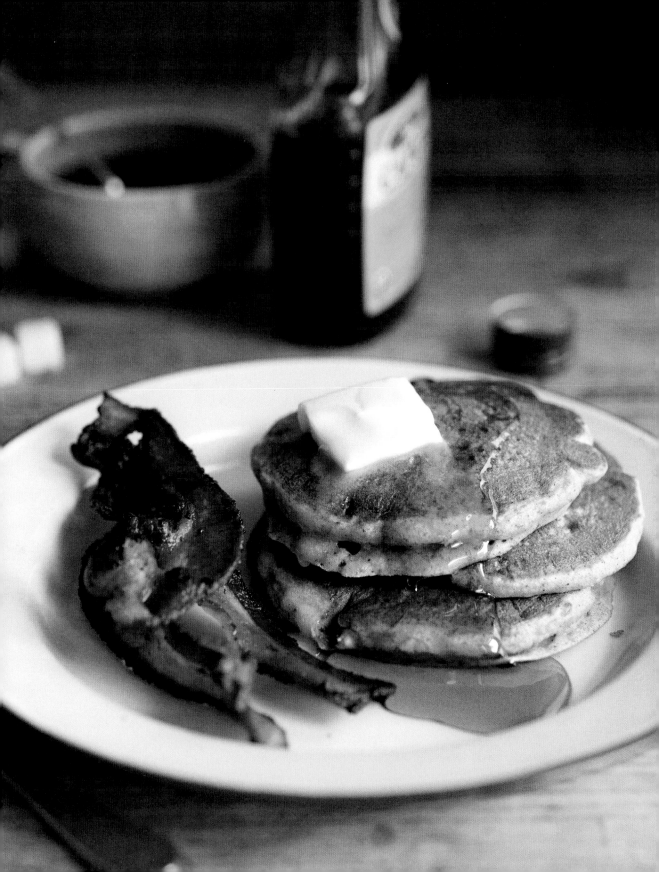

PROTEIN-BOOSTED OATMEAL *with* BERRIES

Morning workout? Consider this meal a bowl full of the nutrition you need. The oatmeal provides a slow-digesting source of carbohydrates, and the jolt of whey powder helps prime your muscle growth for bigger gym gains.

1	cup rolled oats
1	cup 2% milk
½	cup berries (fresh or frozen, your choice of berries)
	Dash of salt
	Dash of ground cinnamon
2	teaspoons honey
1	scoop (28 g) vanilla whey-protein powder

In a large microwaveable bowl, combine the oats and milk. Microwave on high for 1 minute, stir, then microwave for an additional minute. Mix in the berries, salt, cinnamon, and honey. Let the oatmeal cool slightly, then stir in the protein powder. (Very hot oatmeal can damage protein powder, causing it to lump and sour.)

MAKES 1 SERVING · PER SERVING **627** CALORIES // **11 G** FAT // **311 MG** SODIUM // **91 G** CARBOHYDRATES // **10 G** DIETARY FIBER // **43 G** PROTEIN

○ MORE POWER-UPS

Add one or more of these ingredients to your oatmeal for an added shot of nutrients.

2 tablespoons slivered almonds

2 tablespoons golden raisins

1 tablespoon peanut butter

½ banana, sliced

♥

ALMOND PECAN WAFFLES

This recipe swaps in almond flour for wheat flour, giving the waffles a nutty flavor and cutting out the refined carbs. Chopped pecans add another dose of heart-healthy crunch. Serve with pure maple syrup, peanut butter, or fresh fruit.

1	cup almond flour
¼	cup finely chopped pecans
½	cup unflavored whey-protein powder
1	teaspoon baking powder
4	ounces cream cheese, at room temperature
6	eggs
¼	cup heavy cream

1. Preheat a waffle iron.

2. Meanwhile, in a small bowl, combine the almond flour, pecans, whey-protein powder, and baking powder. In another bowl, whisk the cream cheese and 2 of the eggs until smooth. Add the remaining 2 eggs one at a time and whisk thoroughly after each. Mix in the cream, then stir in the dry ingredients.

3. Spoon about ⅓ cup batter onto the hot waffle iron and cook until golden brown, about 3 minutes. Repeat with the remaining batter.

4. Serve right away or let them cool, place in a resealable plastic bag, and freeze. When you're ready to eat one, just pop it in the toaster.

MAKES 6 SERVINGS · PER SERVING **321** CALORIES // **28 G** FAT // **240 MG** SODIUM // **9 G** CARBOHYDRATES // **2.5 G** DIETARY FIBER // **12 G** PROTEIN

EGG, AVOCADO, *and* SPICY MAYO SANDWICH

Drive-thru breakfast foods usually have about as much flavor as the greasy bag they come in. Try this superior breakfast sandwich, created by chef Brian Lockwood of Frasca in Boulder, Colorado. Avocado starts your day off with good fats, and the cayenne-infused mayonnaise will help shake your taste buds awake.

Pinch of cayenne pepper

1 teaspoon mayonnaise

1 whole wheat English muffin

1 egg

1 teaspoon olive oil

3 or 4 slices avocado

Mix the cayenne pepper into the mayonnaise. Split and toast the English muffin and spread each half with the spicy mayo. Heat the oil in a medium skillet over medium heat. Fry the egg until the yolk is still a little bit runny and place it on a muffin half. Top with the avocado and close the sandwich.

MAKES 1 SANDWICH · PER SERVING **354** CALORIES // **22 G** FAT // **354 MG** SODIUM // **30 G** CARBOHYDRATES // **6 G** DIETARY FIBER // **12 G** PROTEIN

○ FLIP A FRIED EGG

CHOOSE THE RIGHT PAN
Go for the medium non-stick variety. A small pan won't leave enough room for both egg and spatula during the flip; a big one may be too heavy to lift.

START COOKING
Melt a tablespoon of butter over medium-low heat. Crack an egg into the pan. When the white is set and no longer jelly-like, it's time to flip.

GIVE IT A SWIRL
Add a few drops of water to the pan and gently swirl. The moisture will help separate the egg from the pan and make the flipping easier.

NOW FLIP!
Tilt the pan at a 45-degree angle and slide the egg onto your spatula. Level the pan and give the spatula a turn to gently flip the egg over without breaking the yolk or doubling the white over.

SMOKED SALMON *and* SCRAMBLED EGGS ON TOAST

Smoked salmon is salty, satisfying, and loaded with omega-3 fatty acids, which have been shown to reduce your risk of heart disease. Plus, it tastes awesome with eggs. Try the combo for yourself with this recipe from Hugh Fearnley-Whittingstall, author of *The River Cottage Fish Book*.

1   slice hearty bread, such as sourdough or whole wheat

2   eggs

    Salt and ground black pepper

1   ounce sliced smoked salmon

    Thinly sliced red onion, capers, chopped fresh dill, and/or a lemon wedge, for serving

Toast the bread. Meanwhile, in a bowl, whisk the eggs with salt and pepper. Pour the eggs into a nonstick pan and scramble them. Lay the smoked salmon on the toast; top that with the scrambled egg. Finish with your choice of red onion, capers, fresh dill, and/or a squeeze of lemon.

MAKES 1 SERVING · PER SERVING 385 CALORIES // 12 G FAT // 756 MG SODIUM // 38 G CARBOHYDRATES // 2 G DIETARY FIBER // 32 G PROTEIN

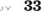

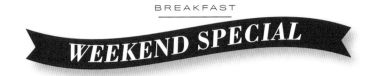

WEEKEND SPECIAL

STUFFED FRENCH TOAST

This is one of the easiest breakfasts that'll show off your cooking chops. You can rustle it up from a few ingredients.

START OFF STALE

Fresh bread has natural moisture that can prevent it from soaking up the egg-milk mixture. Use day-old bread for better absorption, says Candice Kumai, author of *Pretty Delicious,* who provides the step by step for this stuffed French toast. For the best texture, try thick slices of baguette, challah, brioche, or whole wheat bread, or even a split croissant. For this recipe (2 servings), you'll need 4 slices of bread or 2 split croissants.

STACK AND SOAK

Top 2 pieces of bread with one of the "Combos" below. Top with the remaining bread to make 2 sandwiches. In a bowl, whisk 4 eggs with 2 tablespoons milk, 1 teaspoon sugar or maple syrup, and ¼ teaspoon ground cinnamon. Pour into a 13" × 9" baking dish. Place bread stacks in the mixture for 2 minutes, flipping halfway through.

SEAR IT

Melt 1 tablespoon of butter in a medium nonstick skillet over medium-high heat. Place the sandwiches in the pan and cook until golden brown. Serve topped with powdered sugar and whatever fruit you used to stuff the French toast.

COMBO 1:
**Nutella
+
Banana slices**

PER SERVING: 595 CALORIES, 29 G FAT, 458 MG SODIUM, 65 G CARBOHYDRATES, 7 G DIETARY FIBER, 23 G PROTEIN

COMBO 2:
**Cream cheese
+
Raspberries**

PER SERVING: 467 CALORIES, 23 G FAT, 620 MG SODIUM, 47 G CARBOHYDRATES, 4 G DIETARY FIBER, 25 G PROTEIN

COMBO 3:
**Maple syrup
+
Bacon + Apple slices**

PER SERVING: 499 CALORIES, 25 G FAT, 812 MG SODIUM, 45 G CARBOHYDRATES, 5 G DIETARY FIBER, 25 G PROTEIN

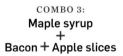

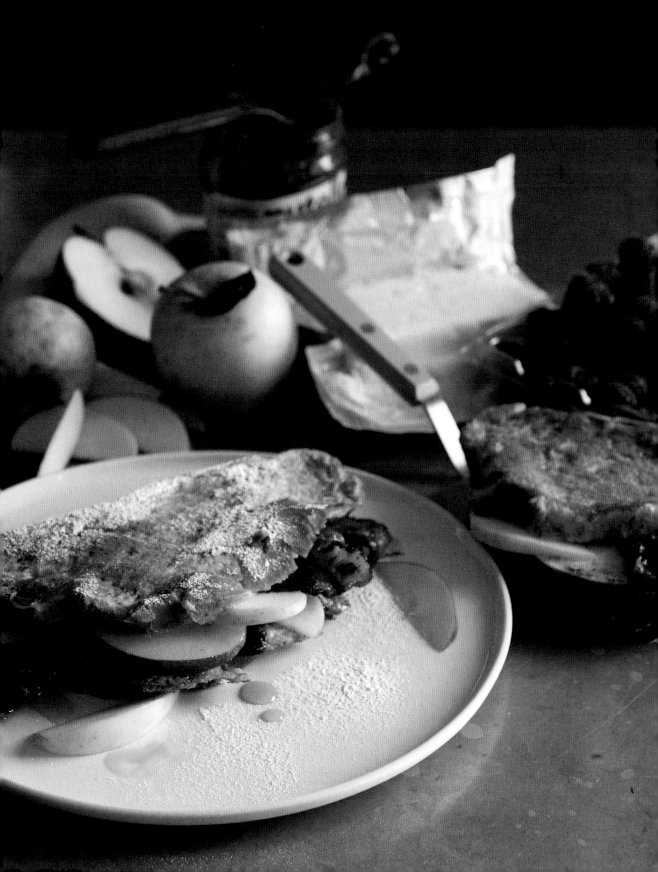

GRANOLA, UPGRADED

A 2011 study published in the *New England Journal of Medicine* links eating whole grains to weight loss. A great all-day source? Granola. Personalize your own heart-healthy, fiber-packed batch. Just be sure to pair it with Greek yogurt for a complementary dose of protein.

START WITH THE BASICS

Preheat the oven to 325°F. Coat a rimmed baking sheet with cooking spray or line it with foil. Add 3 cups of rolled oats and bake until crisp and fragrant, about 20 minutes.

ADD SOME SWEETNESS

Gather up the sticky stuff: In a 1-cup glass measuring cup, stir together ¼ cup apple juice; 3 tablespoons pure maple syrup; 1 tablespoon light brown sugar; 1 tablespoon vegetable oil; ½ teaspoon vanilla extract; and ¼ teaspoon salt.

BAKE IT BROWN

Pour the gooey, sugary mixture over the toasted oats, toss, and bake until crisp and browned, 20 minutes. Allow the granola to cool, and then transfer to a resealable container; seal and store for up to 2 weeks. That's your easy better-than-basic granola recipe. See the add-in options on the next page.

MAKES 6 SERVINGS · PER SERVING **219** CALORIES // **5 G** FAT // **98 MG** SODIUM // **37 G** CARBOHYDRATES // **4 G** DIETARY FIBER // **7 G** PROTEIN

GRANOLA BONUS

For even more nutrition and flavor, add seasonings and ½ cup of chopped nuts to your granola after the first 20 minutes of baking. Then stir in ½ cup of dried fruit after the granola is baked. Here are a few combos to try:

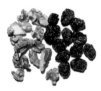

Chopped walnuts
+
Dried cherries
+
Ground ginger
(¾ teaspoon)

PER SERVING: 319 CALORIES, 11 G FAT, 98 MG SODIUM, 47 G CARBOHYDRATES, 7 G DIETARY FIBER, 9 G PROTEIN

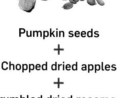

Pumpkin seeds
+
Chopped dried apples
+
Crumbled dried rosemary
(½ teaspoon)

PER SERVING: 299 CALORIES, 10 G FAT, 144 MG SODIUM, 34 G CARBOHYDRATES, 5 G DIETARY FIBER, 10 G PROTEIN

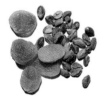

Pistachios
+
Chopped dried apricots
+
Ground cinnamon
(½ teaspoon)
+
Ground cardamom
(½ teaspoon)

PER SERVING: 326 CALORIES, 10 G FAT, 102 MG SODIUM, 51 G CARBOHYDRATES, 7 G DIETARY FIBER, 10 G PROTEIN

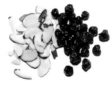

Sliced almonds
+
Dried blueberries
+
Ground allspice
(¼ teaspoon)
+
Ground black pepper
(½ teaspoon)

PER SERVING: 309 CALORIES, 9 G FAT, 102 MG SODIUM, 47 G CARBOHYDRATES, 7 G DIETARY FIBER, 9 G PROTEIN

BETTER BREAKFAST, OVERNIGHT

The Swiss call it muesli— oats soaked in liquid and mixed with fruits and nuts. We just call it good. Sam Talbot, author of *The Sweet Life,* teaches you the technique.

1	cup rolled oats
1	cup water
1	teaspoon honey
½	cup dried cherries and/or raisins
¼	cup chopped walnuts or pecans or sliced almonds
2	tablespoons sunflower seeds
2	tablespoons flaxseeds
1	teaspoon ground cinnamon
1	teaspoon salt
	Plain yogurt, for serving

1. In a bowl, mix together the oats, water, and honey. Soak overnight in the fridge to soften the oats.
2. The following day, stir in the dried fruit, nuts, seeds, cinnamon, and salt. Serve each bowlful topped with a dollop of yogurt.

MAKES 3 SERVINGS

PER SERVING: 335 CALORIES, 14 G FAT, 813 MG SODIUM, 43 G CARBOHYDRATES, 8 G DIETARY FIBER, 10 G PROTEIN

SKILLET EGGS *with* LEEKS *and* ARUGULA

You're ready to go beyond fried and scrambled eggs. Really, you are. Try this simple, impressive dish from *New York Times* food writer Melissa Clark. It pairs over-easy eggs with oniony leeks and assertive arugula, both of which mellow with a little heat.

2	tablespoons butter
2	leeks, thinly sliced
1	clove garlic, finely chopped
	Pinch of salt
8	cups baby arugula
3	tablespoons white wine
	Ground black pepper
4	eggs

1. Melt the butter in a large skillet. Add the leeks and cook until soft. Add the garlic and salt and cook until fragrant. Stir in the arugula and wine and cook until the greens wilt. Season with more salt and some pepper.

2. Crack in the eggs, put the lid on, and cook over low heat until the eggs are lightly set.

MAKES 2 SERVINGS · PER SERVING **339** CALORIES // **22 G** FAT // **339 MG** SODIUM // **18 G** CARBOHYDRATES // **3 G** DIETARY FIBER // **16 G** PROTEIN

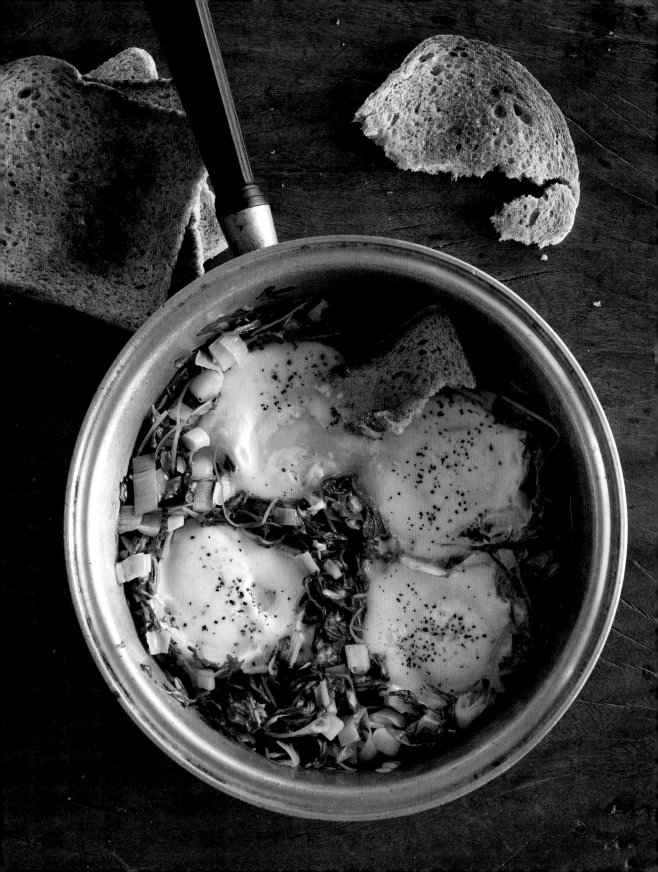

♥

GREEN BURRITO BREAKFAST

No, it's not burritos for beginners. They're green because of the avocados and salsa verde—a smooth salsa made from tomatillos, small, tomato-like fruits that have a bright, acidic bite and are a staple in Mexican cooking.

1½	tablespoons butter
4	eggs, beaten
1½	cups baby spinach
	Salt and ground black pepper
2	corn tortillas
3 or 4	slices avocado
	Salsa verde or tomato salsa

Melt the butter in a nonstick skillet over medium heat. Stir in the eggs and spinach. Season with salt and pepper. Cook, stirring, until the eggs are softly scrambled, about 2 minutes. Wrap the eggs in warm corn tortillas. Top with sliced avocado and salsa verde or tomato salsa.

MAKES 2 SERVINGS · PER SERVING **362** CALORIES // **27 G** FAT // **407 MG** SODIUM // **18 G** CARBOHYDRATES // **6 G** DIETARY FIBER // **16 G** PROTEIN

○ ROLL THE PERFECT BURRITO

This is how you roll your way to better breakfast, lunch, and dinner burritos.

GO BIG
A 12" tortilla lets you stuff your burrito with ingredients yet still provides enough room to wrap it tightly. (Or try a whole wheat wrap for more fiber and a nutty flavor.)

HEAT YOUR TORTILLA
Don't warm tortillas in the microwave—they'll turn soggy. Instead, heat them in a dry skillet or nonstick pan over medium-high until puffed and pliable, 10 to 15 seconds a side.

SET A FOUNDATION
Line the burrito with rice first, to soak up the other ingredients' juices. Next, leaving 3" borders, layer your beans and protein in a vertical line.

APPLY THE FINISHING TOUCHES
Add sour cream, salsa, or guacamole alongside the ingredients. Add loose ingredients (lettuce, cilantro, sliced jalapeños, shredded cheese) last so they can adhere to the sour cream and guac.

LET'S ROLL!
With the line of layered ingredients oriented vertically, fold the tortilla's left side just over the ingredients. Then fold up about 1" of the bottom. Finally, finish rolling the burrito tightly from left to right. One end remains open. Now chow, stain-free.

7 HIGH-SPEED, HIGH-PROTEIN MEALS

Fast doesn't have to mean boring.

Try these creative ways to get out the door with a full belly.

① ITALIAN TOAST

Spread ricotta on whole-grain toast, and top with halved cherry tomatoes, coarse salt, and a drizzle of olive oil.

② FAST RANCHERO

Simmer eggs in your favorite salsa until set. Top with canned black beans and avocado.

③ FIBER PARFAIT

Layer high-fiber cereal, Greek yogurt, berries, and a dash of cinnamon in a bowl.

④ ITALIAN GREENS

Wilt shredded greens (spinach, kale, chard) in olive oil and minced garlic. Crack in eggs and sprinkle with grated Parm, and toss until the eggs are cooked through.

⑤ HEALTHY ELVIS

Toast a slice of hearty whole wheat bread. Spread with a thin layer of crunchy peanut butter, 2 slices of supercrispy bacon, and ½ banana, sliced.

⑥ TOAD IN THE HOLE

In a skillet, heat a slice of whole wheat bread with a circle cut out. Crack an egg into the hole and cook until the egg is set. Sprinkle with salt, pepper, and Tabasco.

⑦ THE BACONATOR

Fry a couple slices of bacon until crisp, then pull the bacon from the pan to drain. Crack a couple eggs into the pan, top with a pile of baby spinach, and cook until eggs are set and greens are wilted. Serve with crispy bacon alongside.

HUEVOS RANCHEROS

Warmed tortillas provide the foundation of this Tex-Mex breakfast.
The yolks of the over-easy eggs on top spill over the rest of the ingredients.
The rich yolk, spicy salsa, and hearty black beans combine to make this
a new go-to in your breakfast repertoire.

1	can (16 ounces) whole peeled tomatoes
½	small onion, chopped
1	clove garlic
1	canned chipotle pepper in adobo sauce, minced (about 1 tablespoon)
¼	cup fresh cilantro sprigs
	Juice of 1 lime
	Salt and ground black pepper
1	can (15 ounces) low-sodium black beans, drained
	Pinch of ground cumin
8	large eggs
8	corn tortillas, warmed

1. In a food processor, combine the tomatoes (with juice), onion, garlic, chipotle pepper, cilantro, and half the lime juice. Pulse until the salsa is well blended but still slightly chunky. Season with salt and black pepper to taste.

2. In a bowl, combine the beans, cumin, and the remaining lime juice. Add salt and black pepper to taste. Use the back of a fork to lightly mash the beans, adding a splash of warm water if the mixture looks dry.

3. Add a shot of cooking spray to a nonstick skillet and heat the pan over medium heat. Crack in the eggs and cook them until the whites have set but the yolks are still runny. In another skillet over medium heat, toast the tortillas about a minute on each side.

4. Spread the beans on the tortillas and top with eggs and salsa. Serve immediately.

MAKES 4 SERVINGS · PER SERVING **390** CALORIES // **13 G** FAT // **573 MG** SODIUM // **52 G** CARBOHYDRATES // **5 G** DIETARY FIBER // **21 G** PROTEIN

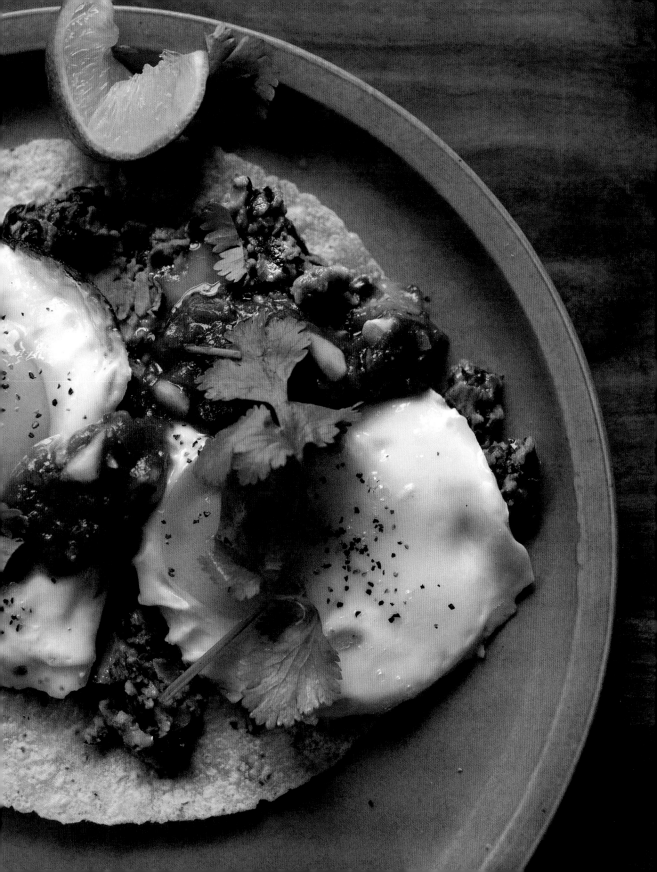

A JAVA WELL DONE

You don't need portion-controlled pods and digital touchscreens to make great coffee at home. "Brewing a single cup with a cone filter is a simple, bullet-proof technique that lets the flavor of the beans shine," says 2010 World Barista Champion Michael Phillips of Chicago's Intelligentsia Coffee & Tea. Follow his method.

THE BEANS

Coffee begins to lose flavor from the moment it's roasted, so find the freshest beans you can, says Phillips. "If there's no roast date on the bag, it may be because the roaster doesn't want you to know it," he says. Find a local roaster, or order online from an artisanal roaster. Aficionados often prefer single-origin brews, but a blend offers a more consistent cup. By mixing beans from several regions, the roaster downplays off-flavors and boosts the best tastes from each bean.

THE GRIND

Exposure to oxygen destroys the volatile oils that give coffee its flavor, so buy your beans whole and grind them yourself. But don't use a spice grinder; it chops unevenly, yielding coffee that's both over- and underextracted. Upgrade to a burr grinder, which pulverizes beans uniformly as they pass through the grinding elements. Models go for as low as $30.

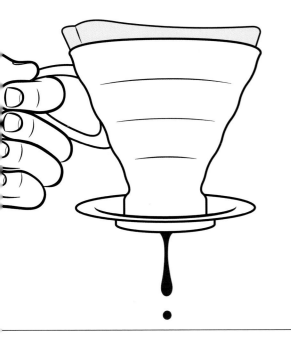

THE CUP

The brightest, cleanest flavor comes from using a simple pour-over cone lined with a paper filter, says Phillips. A bonus: It's easy to clean and takes up almost no counter space. He recommends the Japanese-made Hario V60 02. Store the rest of your beans in an opaque, airtight container at room temperature for up to 2 weeks.

BREW LIKE A BARISTA

STEP 1
HEAT THE WATER

Boiling water can scald the grounds, but water that's too cool won't extract their full flavor. The ideal range is right around 200°F, give or take 5°. To reach that, boil filtered water in a kettle and then let it cool for 30 to 60 seconds.

STEP 2
PREP THE FILTER

Pour a bit of just-boiled water through the filter to saturate it and wash off loose fibers that would sour your coffee. Then toss out any excess water from the cone and place it on top of the mug.

STEP 3
BREW THE COFFEE

Fill the filter with 2 rounded tablespoons of grounds for 8 ounces of brewed coffee. Gradually pour in just enough water to saturate the grounds. Wait for the coffee grounds to "bloom"—60 to 90 seconds. Now, starting in the middle of the cone, pour the water in a slow, narrow stream, working in circles out toward the edge. Don't flood the cone.

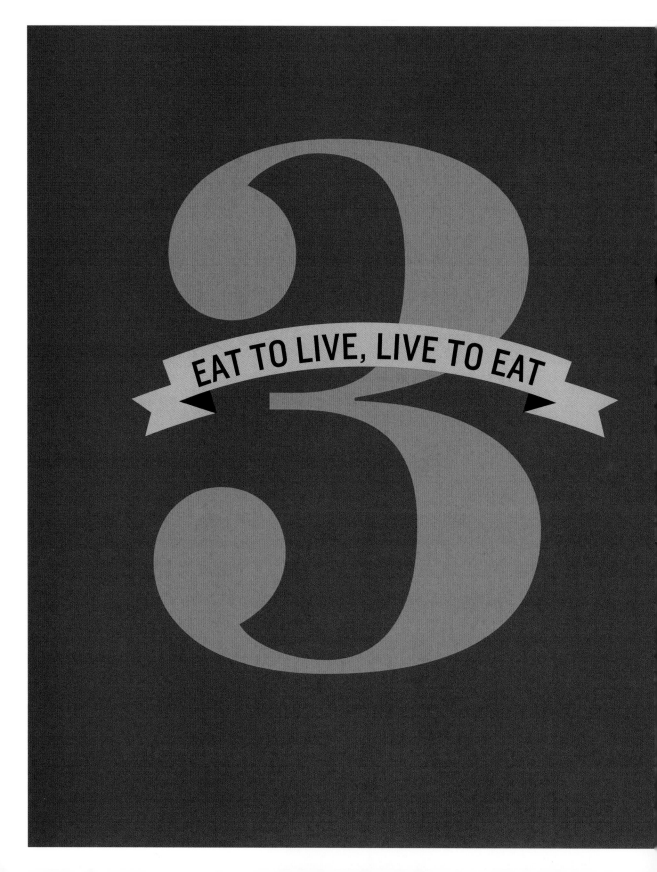

3

EAT TO LIVE, LIVE TO EAT

LUNCH

We've come a long way from the humble PB&J.

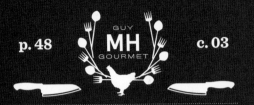

THE RULES *of* LUNCH

By the time you're 25 years old, you will have eaten approximately 9,125 lunches. If you're 40, that's 14,600 lunches. Now, think about this: How many of those lunches have been worth remembering? Not many, eh? Follow these Four Rules of Lunch and you'll avoid a fast-food show-down at high noon and create midday meals worthy of a time out.

RULE Nº.

1

FIND YOUR BALANCE

COME NOON, YOUR brain may crave feel-good carbs—and lots of them—to counteract built-up stress or to reward yourself for a morning of hard work. But give in to a carb binge with a stack of pizza slices or a piled-high sandwich, and you'll crash hard soon after lunch. You want a meal that's high in protein but scores low on the glycemic index—meaning that the carbs it does contain should have little impact on your blood sugar. This keeps your fat-burning furnace stoked and helps prevent a midday lull. So if you go with a sandwich, make sure the bread has at least 3 grams of fiber per slice to help fill you up. Pasta dishes should contain whole grains, too, as should your pizza—but those carb-heavy options are always a poorer choice than more protein-focused fare such as a salmon fillet with a side salad or grilled chicken breast and steamed broccoli.

RULE Nº 2 | CHEW ON THIS

SKIP THOSE SIPPABLE meal-replacement shakes and calorie-clogged smoothies from the juice joint. Thoroughly chewing your food increases what researchers call "oro-sensory factors," which send satiation signals to your brain, helping you feel full on less food, according to a study by Dutch researchers. Study participants who chewed each bite for an extra 3 seconds ended up consuming less.

RULE Nº 3 | LEAN ON LEFTOVERS

YOU CAN TRANSFORM the majority of the recipes in this book into healthy lunches. Grilled meat or seafood can serve as salad mix-ins. Roasted vegetables taste great on sandwiches or wraps. Chili or gumbo buddy-buddy well with brown rice. So when you're packing away extra food from dinner the night before, throw a lunch-size serving into Tupper-ware for the next day's lunch. The limit for pretty much all leftovers is 3 to 4 days. After that, you risk becoming sick from *E. coli*, salmo-nella, and *Staphylococcus aureus*. Exceptions to the bacterial-growth rule are salads with vinegar-based dressings; the dressings contain acids that make it difficult for germs to thrive. In theory, this could extend fridge shelf life. However, those same dressings also make your food soggy after just a day or two.

RULE Nº 4 | LIMIT DISTRACTIONS

WHAT YOU'RE DOING while you eat might be as important as what you're eating. You're likely to consume much more food and eat for longer periods of time when you're distracted by television, music, or a computer, according to a review of studies published in *Trends in Food Science & Technology*. Eating while distracted interrupts brain-to-stomach satiation signals, making it harder to monitor your food intake. Also, distraction raises the risk of overeating the wrong types of foods—think popcorn at the movies. The takeaway from all this is simple: When you eat, actually eat. Grab a seat. Focus on your meal. Don't check your e-mail or hit up Hulu for last night's *The Daily Show*. Pay attention to your first plate of food and you might find that you don't need to go back for seconds.

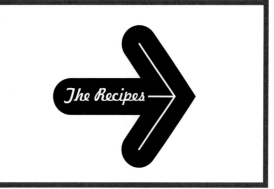

The Recipes →

BUFFALO CHICKEN SANDWICH

If you're craving spicy chicken for lunch, dodge the fast-food joint and opt for this homemade sandwich instead. Its heat comes from hot sauce instead of a spicy fried batter.

½	cup plain Greek yogurt
¼	cup crumbled blue cheese
	Juice of ½ lemon
	Salt and ground black pepper
4	boneless, skinless chicken breast halves (4 to 6 ounces each)
1½	teaspoons chili powder
1	red onion, sliced
2	tablespoons butter, melted in the microwave for 20 seconds
2	tablespoons hot sauce (Frank's RedHot is our pick)
4	romaine lettuce leaves
4	sesame buns, toasted

1. Preheat a grill or nonstick grill pan. As it's heating, combine the yogurt, blue cheese, and lemon juice, plus a pinch each of salt and pepper. Stir and set aside.

2. Season the chicken breasts with the chili powder and salt and pepper to taste. Add the chicken breasts to the hot grill and cook for 5 to 6 minutes on one side before flipping them.

3. Add the onion to the grill's perimeter. (If you're using a grill pan, you'll need to wait to remove the chicken before grilling the onions.) Cook the chicken until firm and springy to the touch, 4 to 5 minutes more. Remove it to a plate, along with the grilled onions.

4. In a small bowl, combine the butter and hot sauce and brush the mixture all over the chicken. Place a leaf of romaine on the bottom half of each bun. Top with a chicken breast and spoon on some blue-cheese sauce. Add grilled onions and the top half of the bun.

MAKES 4 SERVINGS · PER SERVING **421** CALORIES // **16 G** FAT // **680 MG** SODIUM // **25 G** CARBOHYDRATES // **1 G** DIETARY FIBER // **44 G** PROTEIN

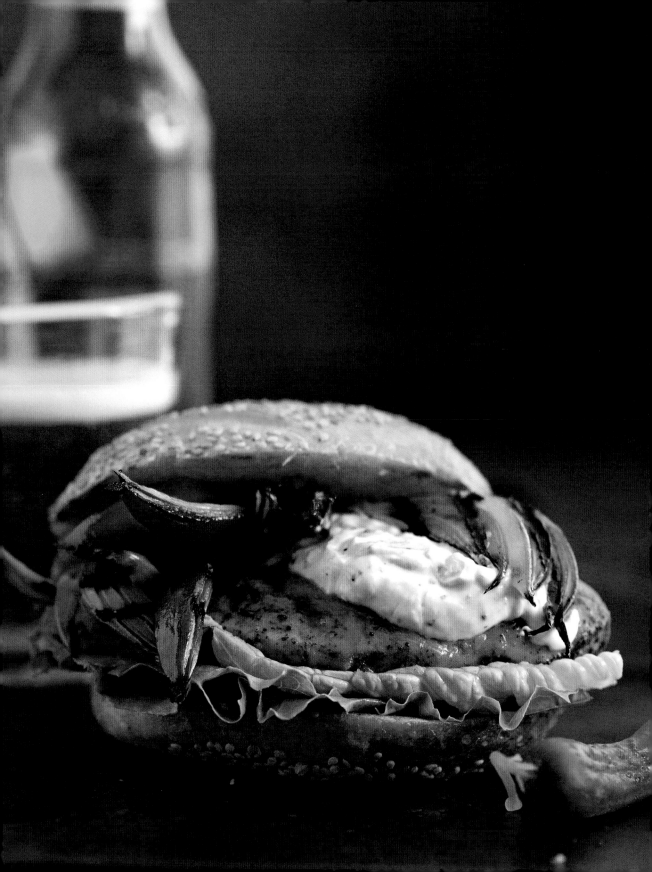

GRILLED CHICKEN *and* PINEAPPLE SANDWICHES

Fired on the grill, pineapple tastes even sweeter, teaming up with the charbroiled flavor of grilled chicken in this satisfying lunch or dinner sandwich.

4	boneless, skinless chicken breast halves (4 to 6 ounces each)
2	tablespoons teriyaki sauce
4	slices Swiss cheese
4	slices pineapple (½" thick)
4	whole wheat kaiser rolls
½	medium red onion, thinly sliced
¼	cup pickled jalapeño slices, or 1 fresh jalapeño chile pepper, thinly sliced

1. Place the chicken in a resealable plastic bag, add enough teriyaki sauce to cover, and let it marinate in the refrigerator for at least 30 minutes (or up to 12 hours).

2. Preheat a grill or grill pan; it's ready when you can't hold your hand above the grate or pan for longer than 5 seconds. Remove the chicken from the marinade and place it on the grill. (Discard any remaining marinade.) Grill for 4 to 5 minutes, flip, and immediately add the cheese to each breast. Continue cooking until the cheese is melted and the chicken is lightly charred and feels firm to the touch. Remove and set aside.

3. While the chicken is resting, place the pineapple slices and rolls on the grill. Toast the rolls lightly and cook the pineapple until it's soft and caramelized, about 2 minutes on each side. Top each roll with chicken and, if you like, drizzle on a bit of teriyaki sauce from the bottle. Top the sandwiches with pineapple, onion, and jalapeño.

MAKES 4 SERVINGS · PER SERVING 392 CALORIES // **13 G** FAT // **744 MG** SODIUM // **33 G** CARBOHYDRATES // **4 G** DIETARY FIBER // **36 G** PROTEIN

VIETNAMESE STEAK SANDWICHES

Philly meets the Far East in this spin on the iconic steak sandwich, developed by Anita Lo, executive chef of Annisa in New York City. Take sliced strip steak, enrobe it in a wrap, and dip it into a spicy-savory Vietnamese sauce and eat up. Sounds crazy, tastes great.

1	**New York strip steak (8 ounces)**
	Salt and ground black pepper
4	**tablespoons canola oil**
2	**tablespoons lime juice**
1	**teaspoon chili garlic sauce, such as Sriracha**
1	**teaspoon fish sauce**
	Pinch of sugar
2	**soft taco-size flour tortillas, warmed**
2	**handfuls of baby greens**
2	**slices red onion**
4	**slices tomato**
½	**avocado, sliced**

1. Heat a skillet or grill pan over medium-high heat. Season the steak with salt and pepper to taste.

2. Add 2 tablespoons of the oil to the pan and cook the steak, turning once, to medium-rare, about 4 minutes per side.

3. In a small bowl, mix together the lime juice, chili garlic sauce, fish sauce, sugar, salt and pepper to taste, and the remaining 2 tablespoons canola oil. Set the sauce aside.

4. Slice the steak and divide the slices between the tortillas. Top each with baby greens, onion, tomato, and avocado. Serve the wraps with the dipping sauce.

PACK IT UP: Store the wraps and dipping sauce separately.

MAKES 2 SERVINGS · PER SERVING **627** CALORIES // **42 G** FAT // **665 MG** SODIUM // **33 G** CARBOHYDRATES // **6 G** DIETARY FIBER // **32 G** PROTEIN

ASIAN BEEF SALAD *with* SRIRACHA HONEY DRESSING

Clobber your salad with creamy dressing and you'll not only ruin a lighter meal, you'll overwhelm the flavors of the greens. Make your own sweet and spicy dressing and use it to top this salad, layered with juicy seared flank steak.

1	pound flank steak
	Salt and ground black pepper
	Juice of 1 lime
2	teaspoons honey
1½	teaspoons lower sodium soy sauce
1	teaspoon Sriracha or other hot sauce
¼	cup canola oil
1	head Bibb lettuce, torn
1	pint cherry tomatoes, halved
1	small red onion, thinly sliced
1	avocado, diced
½	English (hothouse) cucumber, thinly sliced
	Handful of cilantro leaves

1. Preheat a grill, grill pan, or cast-iron skillet over medium-high heat. Season the steak with salt and pepper to taste and cook it to medium-rare, 3 to 4 minutes per side. Let the steak rest for at least 5 minutes and then slice it thinly across the grain.

2. While the meat rests, in a small bowl, whisk together the lime juice, honey, soy sauce, hot sauce, and a pinch of pepper. Gradually whisk in the oil.

3. In a large bowl, toss the steak slices with the vegetables and cilantro. Drizzle in the dressing and toss until the salad is lightly coated.
PACK IT UP: Store the dressing in a separate container and toss it with the salad just before eating.

MAKES 4 SERVINGS · PER SERVING **462** CALORIES // **30 G** FAT // **167 MG** SODIUM // **15 G** CARBOHYDRATES // **5 G** DIETARY FIBER // **34 G** PROTEIN

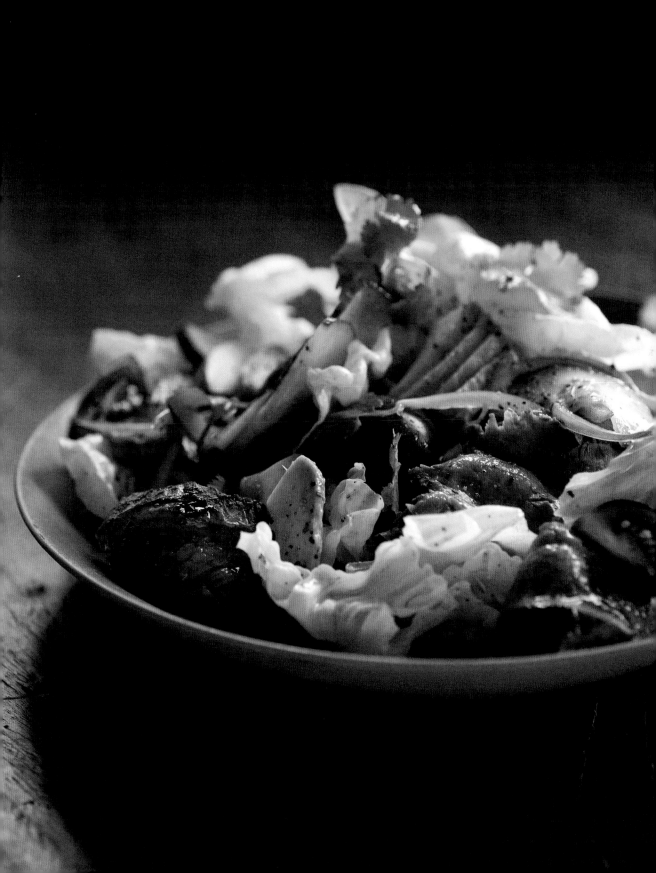

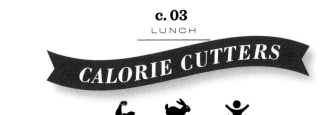

FAST OPEN-FACED SANDWICHES

Consider the open-faced sandwich the convertible of sandwiches. Taking the top off allows you to look good by saving on calories and carbs without skimping on flavor. Wasa crispbread contains just 7 grams of carbs—compared with 21 grams in regular sliced bread. And Kavli crackers are light and wafer-thin, like crispy tortilla pieces. Each rye crisp has only 20 to 40 calories—a sixth of what's in a slice of bread. If you're taking lunch to go, pack the bread and topping separately so the sandwich won't turn soggy before chow time.

PROSCIUTTO ANTIPASTO ON CRISPBREAD

Fresh tomatoes, salty prosciutto, luscious mozzarella—this open-faced sandwich houses enough deliciousness to evoke envy in sandwiches three times its size.

Layer 3 thin slices of prosciutto and some arugula and sliced grape tomatoes on a rye crispbread. Top with a slice of mozzarella cheese and a few drops of olive oil.

PER SERVING: 224 CALORIES, 14 G FAT, 1,133 MG SODIUM, 9 G CARBOHYDRATES, 2 G DIETARY FIBER, 16 G PROTEIN

CURRIED CHICKEN SALAD ON CRISPBREAD

Curry lends a kick to this creamy chicken salad. Spread the mixture on a crispbread for a satisfying crunch that beats the heck out of Wonder Bread.

Mix ¼ cup chopped cooked chicken with 1 tablespoon mayo, ½ rib celery (chopped), ½ teaspoon curry powder, and 1 tablespoon golden raisins. Spoon onto a crispbread.

PER SERVING: 227 CALORIES, 13 G FAT, 165 MG SODIUM, 12 G CARBOHYDRATES, 3 G DIETARY FIBER, 12 G PROTEIN

ROAST BEEF WITH GORGONZOLA

This high-protein, high-fiber, open-faced sandwich goes easy on the carbs, which makes it a lunchtime go-to if you're looking to slim down or stay lean.

Top 1 slice of sprouted whole grain bread with some red onion, 3 slices of roast beef, ¼ cup watercress leaves, and 2 tablespoons creamy Gorgonzola cheese.

PER SERVING: 273 CALORIES, 12 G FAT, 567 MG SODIUM, 18 G CARBOHYDRATES, 4 G DIETARY FIBER, 23 G PROTEIN

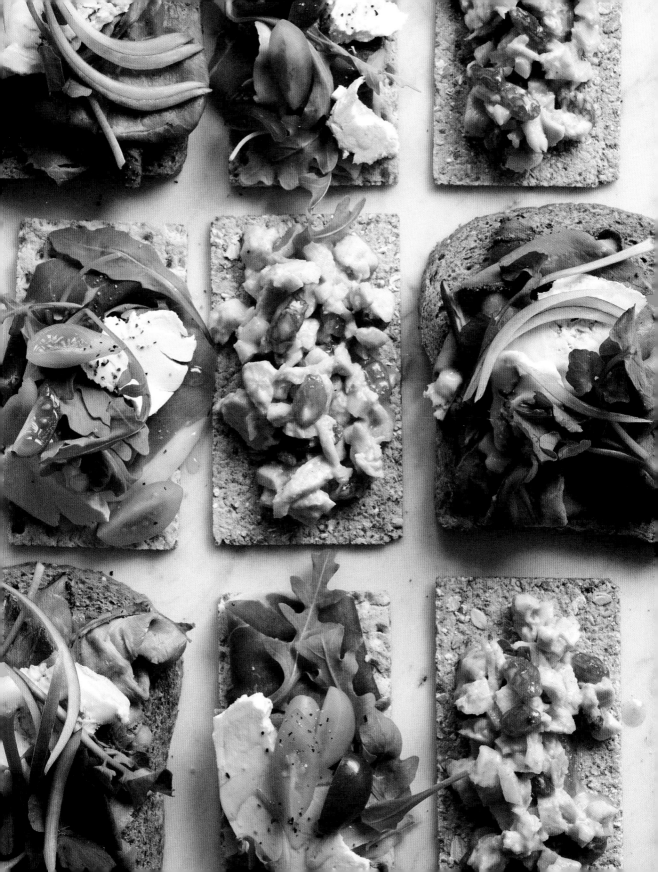

MUSCLE SALAD MATRIX

A daily salad fix can help you stockpile heaps of vital nutrients. Unfortunately, many combos don't offer enough protein and fiber to trigger long-term satiation and fuel muscle growth, says nutritionist Matthew Kadey, M.S., R.D. Plus, he adds, "salad bars can dish out more fat bombs than a Lambeau Field tailgate." Strike the right balance at home with these near-instant meals—all under 550 calories. They all taste great with a simple vinaigrette or one of the dressings on page 61.

NINE GREAT SALAD COMBOS

PROTEIN

HARD-BOILED EGGS +
(2 LARGE EGGS, SLICED)

ROTISSERIE CHICKEN +
(3 OZ SKINNED AND CHOPPED)

SOLID WHITE ALBACORE TUNA +
(3 OZ CANNED, DRAINED AND FLAKED)

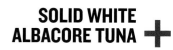

	↓ OPTION 1	↓ OPTION 2	↓ OPTION 3
GREENS	½ head escarole, rinsed and chopped	2 cups arugula	2 cups baby spinach
FLAVOR BOOST	½ cup canned mandarin orange segments, drained	¼ cup dried tart cherries	½ cup fresh blueberries
FIBER	½ cup halved broccoli florets	½ red bell pepper, sliced into strips	½ cup canned lentils, rinsed
TEXTURE	¼ cup pecans	1 oz goat cheese, crumbled	¼ cup walnuts
GREENS	2 cups watercress, stems trimmed	2 cups baby spinach	½ head romaine lettuce, torn
FLAVOR BOOST	½ peach, thinly sliced	¼ cup jarred salsa	½ red apple, diced
FIBER	½ cup halved sugar snap peas	½ cup canned black beans, rinsed	1 celery rib, thinly sliced
TEXTURE	1 oz blue cheese, crumbled	½ avocado, thinly sliced	⅓ cup almonds, chopped
GREENS	½ head Boston lettuce, torn	2 cups thinly sliced kale, ribs removed	2 cups mesclun mix
FLAVOR BOOST	¼ cup niçoise olives	1 Tbsp capers	½ cup jarred roasted red pepper, sliced
FIBER	½ cup canned chickpeas, rinsed	½ cup canned cannellini beans, rinsed	½ cup jarred marinated artichoke hearts
TEXTURE	1 oz smoked mozzarella, cubed	1 oz feta cheese, crumbled	½ avocado, sliced

CALORIE CUTTERS

DO-IT-YOURSELF DRESSINGS

Be careful of most bottled salad dressings. Why? The evidence is right there on the bottle: Just look at the ingredient statement. After soybean oil (a nutritionally inferior fat), you'll likely find a list of thickeners, binders, and preservatives—a bevy of carefully balanced chemicals that form a sludge-like consistency and allow the dressing to survive months without refrigeration. Yum.
You can make a healthier dressing that tastes a whole lot better than any in a bottle. And it'll take you less than 5 minutes. Your payoff will be more flavor, more health-promoting ingredients, and calorie savings. Oh, you'll save money, too.

o WHY NOT MAKE A NONFAT DRESSING?

You could cut more calories by using fat-free mayonnaise and yogurt, but that would be a mistake. Researchers from Ohio State University found that adding fat to salad increased the body's ability to absorb nutrients. Even the smallest amount of fat tested increased lutein and beta-carotene absorption by more than 400 percent.

HERE'S HOW TO DRESS BETTER INSTANTLY:

For all dressings, combine the ingredients in a medium bowl and stir until uniform. They all make 6 servings.

BLUE CHEESE

BOTTLED STANDARD:

Wishbone Chunky Blue Cheese (2 tablespoons): 150 calories

MAKE IT YOURSELF:

- ¼ cup 2% plain Greek yogurt
- 2 tablespoons olive-oil mayonnaise
- 2 tablespoons water
- 1 tablespoon white wine vinegar
- ¼ teaspoon ground black pepper
- **Pinch of cayenne pepper**
- ¼ cup crumbled blue cheese

Refrigerate for up to 2 weeks.

POUR IT ON:

BEST GREENS: romaine or iceberg

BEST TOPPINGS: grape tomatoes, carrots, and celery

PER 2-TABLESPOON SERVING: 45 CALORIES, 4 G FAT, 121 MG SODIUM, 1 G CARBOHYDRATES, 1 G DIETARY FIBER, 2 G PROTEIN

HONEY MUSTARD

BOTTLED STANDARD:

Marie's Honey Mustard (2 tablespoons): 140 calories

MAKE IT YOURSELF:

- ½ cup spicy brown mustard
- 2 tablespoons honey
- 1 tablespoon water
- 2 teaspoons lemon juice
- 2 teaspoons olive oil

Refrigerate for up to 3 months.

POUR IT ON:

BEST GREENS: shredded cabbage or Boston lettuce

BEST TOPPINGS: carrots, broccoli, and sugar snap peas

PER 2-TABLESPOON SERVING: 56 CALORIES, 2 G FAT, 202 MG SODIUM, 6 G CARBOHYDRATES, 0 G DIETARY FIBER, 0 G PROTEIN

CAESAR

BOTTLED STANDARD:

Ken's Creamy Caesar (2 tablespoons): 170 calories

MAKE IT YOURSELF:

- 6 tablespoons olive-oil mayonnaise
- 3 tablespoons lemon juice
- 2 tablespoons water
- 6 anchovy fillets, mashed, or 2 teaspoons anchovy paste
- ⅓ cup grated Parmesan cheese

Refrigerate for up to 1 month.

POUR IT ON:

BEST GREENS: romaine or radicchio

BEST TOPPINGS: sliced mushrooms and asparagus

PER 2-TABLESPOON SERVING: 65 CALORIES, 5 G FAT, 284 MG SODIUM, 1 G CARBOHYDRATES, 0 G DIETARY FIBER, 3 G PROTEIN

PILLAGE THE FARMERS' MARKET
Find freshness close to home.

These days, farmers' markets are popping up faster than dandelions on an herbicide-free lawn. Here's how to shop smart and come back with the best.

1
SET YOUR ALARM

The sweetest strawberries, crispest cucumbers, and most vibrant greens are often snatched up in the first hour the market is open, so it pays to arrive early to score the cream of the crop. The vendors have more time to chat then, too, so ask them which fruits and vegetables are at peak ripeness.

2
SHOOT FOR THE RAINBOW

For the widest variety of antioxidants, select as many differently hued fruits and vegetables as you can stuff into your canvas tote. (You have one of those, right?) Cell-protecting antioxidants are what give many fruits and vegetables their bright colors, and by mixing it up, you ensure you're consuming the entire arsenal.

3
TRY A PURPLE CARROT

Some of the more unfamiliar fruits and vegetables are also among the most flavorful and nutritious. And buying them at a farmers' market probably means you pay less for them than you would at a tony gourmet market. So when you see fresh currants, purple carrots, rainbow chard, and spiky kohlrabi, don't walk past. Ask the vendor how to cook it, and then take it home.

4
EMBRACE UGLY DUCKLINGS

Big produce growers often prioritize pleasant, uniform appearance—not flavor. The oddest-looking varieties of tomatoes and plums at markets can be the best tasting, and they may cost less too.

5
DON'T BE SHY

If you're trying to avoid fruits and vegetables that were swimming in pesticides, look the farmer in the eye and ask how the produce was grown. Many farms use organic practices but don't take the trouble to become certified because of cost or paperwork.

6
SHOP AROUND

Since a range of vendors are often selling the same assortment of produce, be prudent and take a lap around the market before buying anything. Check prices and take a closer look at the wares; you'll probably start to find vendors you prefer.

7
FREEZE EXTRAS

When local raspberries, peaches, and kale are abundant at friendly prices, be sure to freeze some for winter, when you're forced to rely on meager produce-aisle offerings. Many market stands offer discounts for bulk purchases.

GAZPACHO CHOPPED SALAD
with FRESH MOZZARELLA
and PROSCIUTTO

Probably the most famous uncooked summer soup becomes a
main-dish salad here, enhanced with chewy fresh mozzarella and thinly
sliced prosciutto. To make homemade croutons, toast stale white
bread for 10 minutes.

⅔ cup cubed unsalted fresh mozzarella

1 clove garlic

2 cups plain crustless white-bread croutons, store-bought or homemade

2 tablespoons finely chopped roasted piquillo peppers

1½ tablespoons sherry vinegar

1 cup chopped cucumber

1 large tomato, roughly chopped

½ teaspoon kosher salt

1 teaspoon red wine vinegar

⅓ cup olive oil

4 slices prosciutto, roughly torn

1. On a plate, very lightly salt the chopped mozzarella. On a cutting board or in a mortar and pestle, slice and pound the garlic to a paste, adding a little salt.

2. In a bowl, combine the croutons, garlic paste, peppers, and sherry vinegar. Mix well and let sit for 5 minutes.

3. Meanwhile, in another bowl, combine the cucumber, tomato, half the salt, and red wine vinegar. Once the croutons have begun to soften, combine the contents of the two bowls. Add the olive oil, mozzarella, and prosciutto. Taste for salt, adjusting if needed. Serve on 2 plates, drizzled with more olive oil if you like.

MAKES 2 SERVINGS · PER SERVING **648** CALORIES // **50 G** FAT // **1,531 MG** SODIUM // **28 G** CARBOHYDRATES // **3 G** DIETARY FIBER // **20 G** PROTEIN

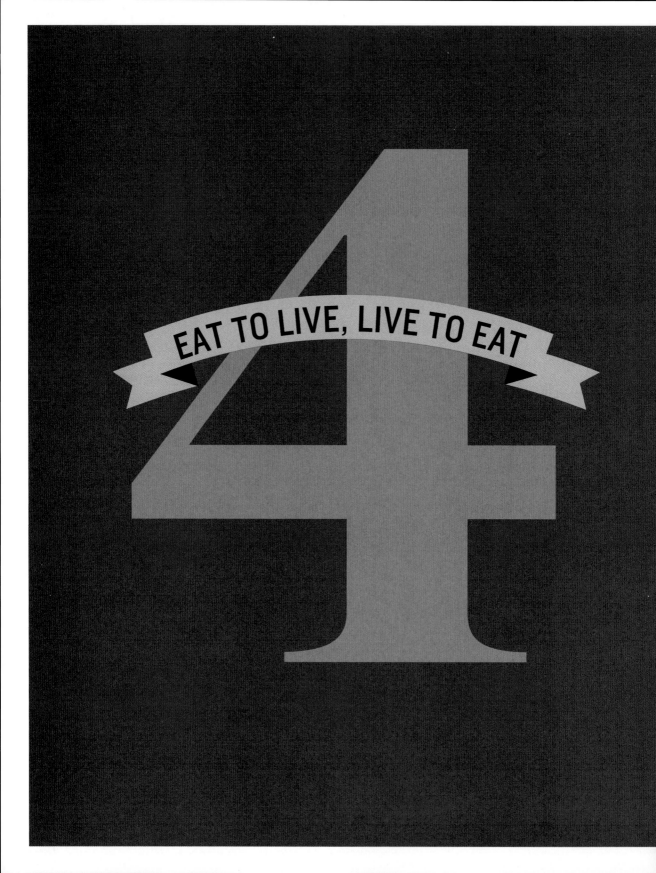

MUSCLE SNACKS

Refuel in between main meals to keep your brain and body humming and your fat-burners stoked.

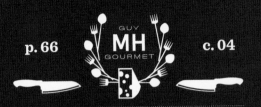

MAKE YOUR SNACKS MEAN SOMETHING

The puffed cheese curl serves no higher purpose than to color your fingertips and make you thirsty.

If you're craving something crunchy and orange, you'd be better off eating popcorn while wearing polarized sunglasses. Snacks should be tasty, but you can make them count for much more with these simple rules.

RULE Nº.

1

MANAGE YOUR HUNGER

SNACKS CAN BE amazing weight-loss tools, bridging the gap between your main meals. By choosing right, you can use snacks to regulate your blood sugar to avoid becoming weak with hunger and eating voraciously at mealtimes, consuming too many calories. The problem is that most store-bought snack foods aren't designed to do that. They are loaded with empty calories and chemicals (did you know there are more than 18 ingredients in Cheetos?) that do nothing for you but trigger more cravings. Gain control by making your own snack foods, incorporating satiating protein, fat, and fiber-rich, slow-burning carbohydrates like those found in fruits, vegetables, and whole grains.

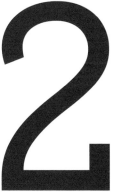

BOOKEND WORKOUTS WITH PROTEIN

EVERY TIME YOU DO resistance exercises, your muscles tear and break down. That makes them primed to respond to protein, says Jeffrey Volek, Ph.D., R.D., a researcher at the University of Connecticut. "You have a window of opportunity to promote muscle growth." Eating protein before and after a workout will provide a fresh infusion of amino acids to repair and build new muscle. Have a turkey or ham sandwich before you work out, and down a whey protein smoothie (recipes start on page 84) right after your workout to speed the protein and carbs into your muscles.

RULE N<u>o</u>

3 SNACK SMART AT WORK

SNACKS ARE ALL about convenience and portability, which is what makes them perfect office supplies. Instead of running to the vending machine or snagging a doughnut, reach into your desk drawer for a handful of raw almonds from your stash. Or slather an apple or banana with natural peanut butter. Bring a small cooler with deli turkey breast to roll around a low-fat cheese stick. Shoot for a total of 10 to 20 grams of protein with a little fat, and you'll stifle cravings until mealtime.

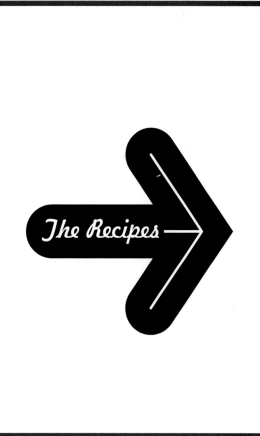

The Recipes →

QUICK SNACK COMBOS

GUAC, ROAST BEEF, *and* SWISS ROLL-UP

In a rush? Turn to this superfast, no-carb snack. For even more flavor, instead of buying a tub of store-bought guacamole, make your own using the recipe on page 149.

Spread a dollop of guacamole on a slice of roast beef, and then roll the roast beef up in a slice of Swiss cheese. Secure with a toothpick. Make a batch and serve them on game day.

PER ROLL-UP: 176 CALORIES, 21 G PROTEIN

ARTICHOKES, ROASTED RED PEPPERS, OLIVES, *and* PARMESAN CHEESE PLATE

Assemble this medley of Mediterranean ingredients along with a good-quality Parmesan for an afternoon or evening snack that's low in calories but high in flavor.

Arrange marinated artichoke hearts, roasted red peppers, and good olives on a platter with a chunk of real Parmesan (or Manchego or Gruyère) and a thin slice of nice ham.

PER 2 PIECES EACH OF ARTICHOKE, PEPPER, AND CHEESE, PLUS 4 OLIVES AND 1 SLICE OF HAM: 202 CALORIES, 12 G PROTEIN

WATERMELON, CHERRY TOMATOES, FRESH MOZZARELLA, *and* PESTO SKEWERS

Trust us on this one. The instant appetizer tastes best in late summer when watermelon and cherry tomatoes are at their peaks.

Thread chunks of watermelon, cherry tomatoes, small balls of fresh mozzarella, and a few basil leaves on wooden skewers. It's summer on a stick.

PER 2 TOMATOES, 2 CHUNKS OF MELON, AND 1 CHEESE BALL: 134 CALORIES, 8 G PROTEIN

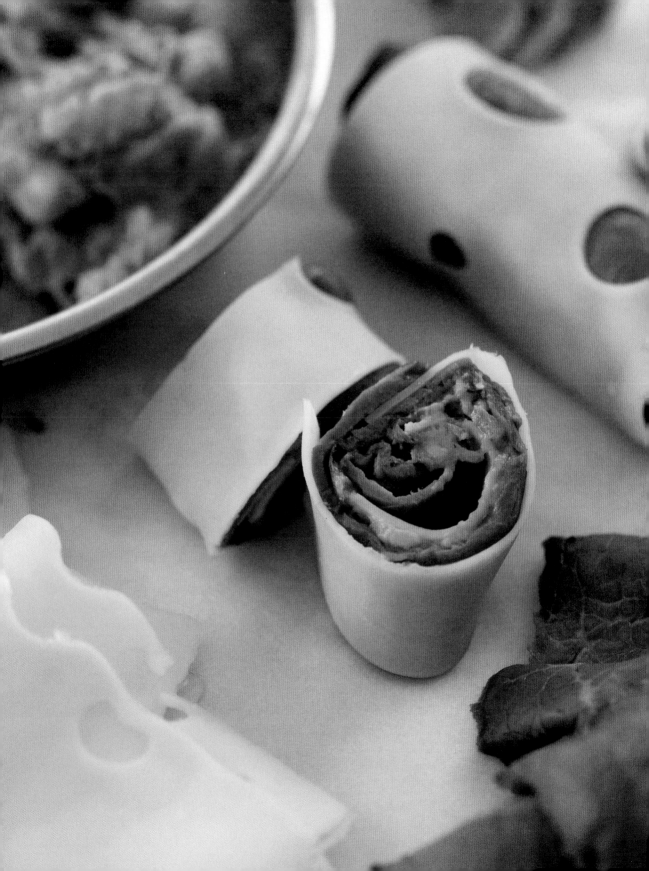

BABA GHANOUSH
with PITA CHIPS

Love hummus? Then you'll also like this smooth, creamy dip that's made from roasted eggplant. Scoop it with a handful of pita chips.

PER 8 CHIPS: 205 CALORIES, 4 G PROTEIN

EGG SALAD LETTUCE WRAP

Skip the bread and you'll cut carbs. Just make sure you choose a sturdy lettuce to carry the heft of the egg salad.

Chop two hard-boiled eggs and mix with diced pickles, a spoon of olive-oil mayonnaise, spicy mustard, and a pinch of cayenne. Spoon the egg salad onto romaine or Bibb lettuce and eat like a burrito.

PER 2 EGGS: 210 CALORIES, 13 G PROTEIN

HONEY WITH GREEK YOGURT *and* FIG

Greek yogurt tastes sour by nature, but its flavor works well when you add in ingredients that deliver a dose of mellow sweetness. Eat this as a healthy postworkout snack or as an easy dessert.

Drizzle 1 teaspoon honey into a cup of 2% Greek yogurt and eat with a fig.

PER CUP: 224 CALORIES, 17 G PROTEIN

PROSCIUTTO-WRAPPED MELON

Make up a batch of these salty-sweet, two-ingredient appetizers for an easy summer snack or a take-along to a buddy's backyard barbecue.

Wrap a strip of prosciutto or good Spanish ham around a slice of honeydew melon or cantaloupe and top with cracked black pepper.

PER WRAPPED SLICE: 88 CALORIES, 5 G PROTEIN

PIZZA MUFFINS

Cut back on your carbs and still have your pizza fix with these fast-bake mini-pies. Use them to fight off late-night snack attacks. This makes 4 muffin halves, but you can save the leftovers and reheat later.

Preheat the oven to 425°F. Spread 2 tablespoons pesto on 4 English muffin halves. Divide 4 tablespoons goat cheese, 2 tablespoons chopped green or kalamata olives, and 4 water-packed artichoke hearts (quartered) among the muffins. Place the muffins on a baking sheet and bake until the cheese is melted and the bottoms are slightly crisp, about 5 minutes.

PER MUFFIN HALF: 157 CALORIES, 6 G PROTEIN

SPICY ROASTED CHICKPEAS

When cooked in the oven, chickpeas crisp up and develop a satisfying crunch. The earthy spices in this recipe only enhance their flavor.

2	cups canned chickpeas, rinsed and drained
1½	teaspoons extra-virgin olive oil
½	teaspoon ground cumin
½	teaspoon ground coriander
¼	teaspoon ground red pepper
¼	teaspoon ground black pepper

1. Preheat the oven to 400°F. Coat a nonstick baking sheet with cooking spray and set aside.

2. In a small bowl, toss the chickpeas with the oil, cumin, coriander, red pepper, and black pepper.

3. Place the chickpeas in a single layer on the baking sheet. Bake for 30 to 40 minutes, or until crisp and golden.

MAKES 8 SERVINGS · PER SERVING **80** CALORIES // **2 G** FAT // **180 MG** SODIUM // **14 G** CARBOHYDRATES // **3 G** DIETARY FIBER // **3 G** PROTEIN

○ TWEAK THE HEAT

1 Southwest Roasted Chickpeas.
Replace the coriander with chili powder.

2 Cajun Roasted Chickpeas.
Replace the cumin, coriander, red pepper, and black pepper with 1 teaspoon Cajun spice.

SPICY OVEN FRIES

Put away the deep fryer and experience healthier, tastier spuds with this baking method.

4	russet potatoes, cut lengthwise into 12 wedges
2	egg whites, lightly beaten
1	teaspoon chili powder
1	teaspoon ground cumin
1	teaspoon paprika
1	teaspoon dried oregano
¼	teaspoon dried thyme
1	teaspoon salt
⅛	teaspoon ground red pepper

1. Preheat the oven to 450°F. Coat a baking sheet with cooking spray. Dip the cut potatoes in the egg to coat and place in a bowl. Mix the remaining ingredients and sprinkle over the potatoes. Toss well to coat.

2. Place the wedges on the baking sheet. Bake for 20 minutes. Turn the potatoes over and bake for 15 minutes or until crisp.

MAKES 4 SERVINGS · PER SERVING **183** CALORIES // **1 G** FAT // **627 MG** SODIUM // **40 G** CARBOHYDRATES // **4 G** DIETARY FIBER // **7 G** PROTEIN

SMOKY PAPRIKA KALE CHIPS

Baking kale draws out its water content, causing it to crisp. Crunch this smoky-salty snack and you could quell your yen for potato chips.

1	large bunch kale
¼	cup olive oil
1	tablespoon smoked paprika
½	teaspoon sea salt

1. Preheat the oven to 400°F. Remove the tough stems from the kale and wash and tear the leaves into large pieces. In a large bowl, toss the kale pieces with the olive oil and paprika.

2. Line a baking sheet with parchment paper, scatter the kale atop, and roast until the greens are dry and crispy, about 30 minutes, tossing every 10 minutes to toast evenly. Toss with the sea salt and serve.

MAKES 6 SERVINGS · PER SERVING **150** CALORIES // **10 G** FAT // **255 MG** SODIUM // **14 G** CARBOHYDRATES // **3 G** DIETARY FIBER // **5 G** PROTEIN

MIX UP A TRAIL SNACK

Long hikes require nutritionally balanced fuel, with enough
energy to sustain prolonged exercise, but not enough to weigh you down.
Bypass the candy posing as "granola bars" at the grocery store
and make this recipe from Devon Metz, R.D., founder of Fit Health
into Life at Devon Hiking Spa, in Boulder, Colorado.

TOSS THESE TOGETHER IN A PLASTIC BAGGIE TO MIX.

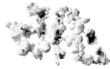

2 CUPS POPCORN

Complex carbs equal energy; fiber fills you up.

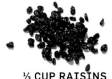

⅓ CUP RAISINS

Raisins' iron content boosts oxygen delivery.

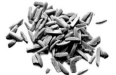

3 TABLESPOONS RAW ALMOND SLIVERS

Monounsaturated fats provide long-lasting energy.

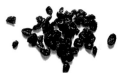

⅓ CUP DRIED CRANBERRIES

Cranberries house antioxidants and have
antibacterial properties.

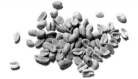

3 TABLESPOONS PEANUTS

Peanuts contribute protein, healthy fats, and
L-arginine, an amino acid that helps control bloodflow.

CINNAMON TO TASTE

Cinnamon flavors the mix without relying on the
salt many prepackaged mixes contain.

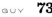

MAKES 4 SERVINGS · PER SERVING **152** CALORIES // **6 G** FAT // **2 MG** SODIUM // **24 G** CARBOHYDRATES //
3 G DIETARY FIBER // **4 G** PROTEIN

5 PROTEIN-PACKED GYM SNACKS

1

DELI CHICKEN OR TURKEY, OR CANNED TUNA
(3 ounces)

14–22 grams protein, 66–100 calories

Wrap one of these standbys in a piece of whole wheat bread. Four slices of chicken or turkey provide 14 grams of protein, while half a can of tuna has nearly 22 grams.

2

EGGS
(3)

19 grams protein, 232 calories

They're still incredible after all these years. Hard-boiled eggs are most convenient, but it's also easy to scramble a few in the a.m. and scoop them into a microwaveable container. Don't sweat the fat: It's healthy and filling.

3

CHOCOLATE 2% MILK
(16 ounces)

17 grams protein, 333 calories

Refresh and rebuild at the same time. A study in the *Journal of the American College of Nutrition* shows that chocolate milk may be the ideal postworkout beverage for building muscle.

4

PROTEIN SHAKE
(with a 30-gram scoop of protein powder)

24 grams protein, 110 calories

Mix it with milk instead of water if you want a bit more protein. Try Nitrean; it has whey isolate for quick absorption, and casein, which is digested slowly so it builds muscle on two fronts.

5

GREEK YOGURT
(6-ounce container)

12 grams protein, 130 calories

Greek yogurt is a lifter's dream: It's easy to carry and packed with protein. Skip yogurts with fruit and sugar; to add flavor, drop in a few berries or nuts.

○ SKIP THE SNACK ADS

Your DVR can help you lose weight. A Yale University study found that people who watched TV commercials advertising snacks ate more cookies and snack mix immediately afterward than those who saw other kinds of ads.

ROSEMARY BAR NUTS

Addictive little buggers, those beer nuts, aren't they? Make a batch for your next game day and pair with—what else—beer.

2   egg whites
3½ tablespoons light brown sugar
¼   teaspoon salt
⅛   teaspoon ground red pepper
    Leaves from 1 large rosemary sprig, chopped
2¼ cups raw mixed nuts

1. Preheat the oven to 300°F. In a large bowl, mix the egg whites, brown sugar, salt, red pepper, and rosemary into a thick paste. Add the nuts and toss until they're coated.

2. Spread the nuts on a sheet pan lined with parchment paper and roast for 20 minutes, tossing every 5 minutes. Transfer to a cold pan and let cool. Store at room temp in an airtight container up to 1 week.

MAKES 8 SERVINGS · PER SERVING **208** CALORIES // **16 G** FAT // **83 MG** SODIUM // **12 G** CARBOHYDRATES // **2 G** DIETARY FIBER // **7 G** PROTEIN

CHOCOLATE-COVERED PRETZELS

Need to satisfy your salty-sweet jones? Make this superfast snack.

2   tablespoons semisweet chocolate chips
2   tablespoons cashews, chopped
3   pretzel rods

Place the chocolate chips in a large, flat microwaveable bowl or plate and microwave until melted (oven power varies, so microwave in 20-second increments). Place the cashews on a second plate. Roll one end of each pretzel rod in the chocolate followed by the cashews. Let cool until firm.

MAKES 1 SERVINGS · PER SERVING **309** CALORIES // **15 G** FAT // **615 MG** SODIUM // **41 G** CARBOHYDRATES // **3 G** DIETARY FIBER // **7 G** PROTEIN

BETTER-FOR-YOU BEEF JERKY

The problem with store-bought jerky is that it's often too salty and laden with chemical additives. Use your oven to cook up a healthier jerky using this recipe from John Schenk, executive chef of Strip House in New York City.

3	**pounds strip steak, trimmed of all visible fat**
5	**tablespoons dark brown sugar**
4	**cloves garlic, chopped**
2	**tablespoons rice vinegar**
3	**tablespoons oyster sauce**
3	**tablespoons soy sauce**
1	**tablespoon ground coriander**
1½	**teaspoons curry powder**
	Juice of 1 lime
	A few chopped cilantro leaves

1. Start by putting the strip steak in the freezer for 3 minutes to make it easier to slice.

2. Use a long, sharp knife to cut the strip steak in half lengthwise, then again crosswise. Then cut it lengthwise into thin strips. Use a meat pounder to lightly flatten the strips to ⅛" thick.

3. In a medium bowl, make a marinade by whisking together the brown sugar, garlic, rice vinegar, oyster sauce, soy sauce, coriander, curry powder, lime juice, and cilantro. Place the beef in a large resealable plastic bag, add the marinade, and leave in the fridge for at least 4 hours or up to a day.

4. Preheat the oven to 200°F. Place the slices on a wire rack set over a baking sheet. Bake until dry, about 45 minutes.

MAKES 8 SERVINGS · PER SERVING **439** CALORIES // **27 G** FAT // **613 MG** SODIUM // **11 G** CARBOHYDRATES // **0 G** DIETARY FIBER // **36 G** PROTEIN

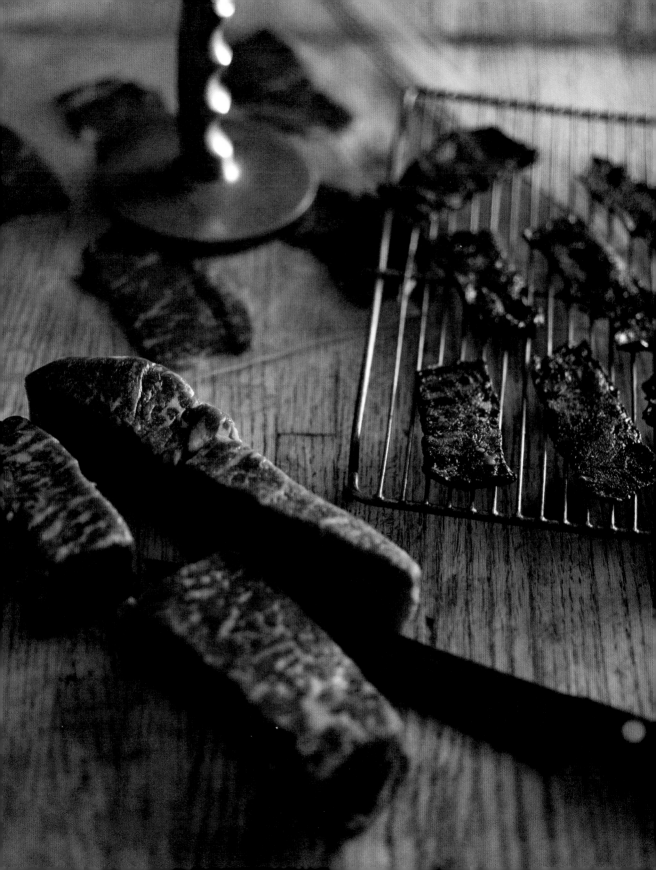

SALUTE THE KERNEL!

Popcorn contains 15 times the disease-fighting polyphenols of whole-grain tortilla chips, according to a recent University of Scranton study. The reason: Unlike corn tortilla chips, popcorn includes the nutrient-packed hull of the corn kernel. Use the stovetop, not a microwave, for fresher-tasting, more thoroughly popped kernels, says Aida Mollenkamp, host of the Food Network's *Ask Aida*.

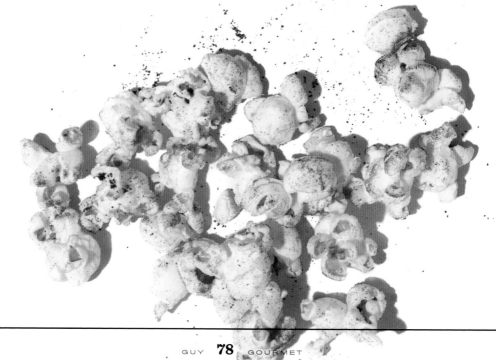

1 PREP YOUR POT

In a large pot, heat 2 tablespoons canola oil and a few popcorn kernels over medium-high heat. When the kernels begin to pop, the oil is hot enough. Remove the pot from the heat and add ¼ cup popcorn kernels and ½ teaspoon kosher salt. Put on the lid and count to 20, off the heat, allowing the popcorn and oil to reach the same temperature; otherwise some of the kernels will burn.

2 STEAM AND SHIMMY

Move the pot back onto the burner and then, with one hand, gently move the pot back and forth over the burner; with your other hand, hold the lid like a shield over the pot, leaving it slightly ajar. The idea is to let the steam escape without letting the popcorn kernels leap out. Heat the popcorn until you notice a delay of several seconds between pops, about 3 minutes total.

3 COAT THE KERNELS

In a small pot, melt 2 tablespoons unsalted butter and, if you want, add additional flavors. Dump the popcorn into a large bowl. Once the butter is melted, pour it over the popcorn, cover the bowl with a dinner plate, and give it a few shakes to coat evenly. Serve immediately.

MAKES 5 TO 6 CUPS POPCORN, OR 3 SERVINGS

PER SERVING **207** CALORIES // **18 G** FAT // **322 MG** SODIUM // **11 G** CARBOHYDRATES // **2 G** DIETARY FIBER // **2 G** PROTEIN

SUPERIOR SEASONINGS

SWEET BOMBAY

2 teaspoons hot Madras curry powder

+

2 teaspoons sugar

+

¾ cup toasted flaked unsweetened coconut

SALT RIM MARGARITA

1 tablespoon tequila

+

2 teaspoons chopped pickled jalapeños

+

1 minced clove garlic

+

zest and juice from 1 lime

CAESAR CROUTON FLAVOR

¼ cup grated Parmesan

+

1 teaspoon fresh thyme leaves

+

1 minced clove garlic

+

½ teaspoon ground black pepper

SNACK MATRIX

Hundred-calorie snack packs are the hottest thing in the packaged food industry since the hot sauce wars of '87. But while they may provide a decent defense against portion distortion, nearly all of them are total junk. Why not make your own instead?

KEY:

- FIBER
- PROTEIN
- HEALTHY FAT

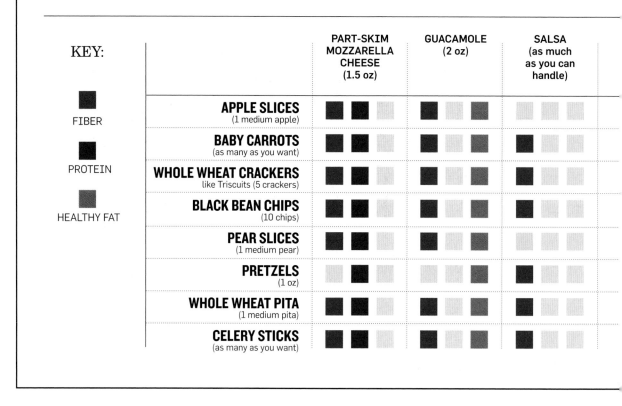

	PART-SKIM MOZZARELLA CHEESE (1.5 oz)	GUACAMOLE (2 oz)	SALSA (as much as you can handle)
APPLE SLICES (1 medium apple)			
BABY CARROTS (as many as you want)			
WHOLE WHEAT CRACKERS like Triscuits (5 crackers)			
BLACK BEAN CHIPS (10 chips)			
PEAR SLICES (1 medium pear)			
PRETZELS (1 oz)			
WHOLE WHEAT PITA (1 medium pita)			
CELERY STICKS (as many as you want)			

Each component adds up to 100 calories, which is ideal since two 200-calorie snacks, strategically timed throughout the day, are just what your body needs to maximize metabolism and keep you burning calories around the clock.

More than anything, you'll see how easy it is to put together a great-tasting combo loaded with the foundations of sound snacking: fiber, lean protein, healthy fat, and a cache of nutrients, or some delicious combination thereof. If the box is empty, it's because the foods don't go well together.

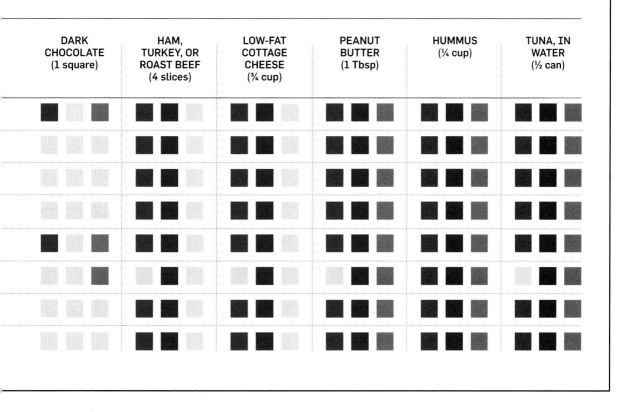

| DARK CHOCOLATE (1 square) | HAM, TURKEY, OR ROAST BEEF (4 slices) | LOW-FAT COTTAGE CHEESE (¾ cup) | PEANUT BUTTER (1 Tbsp) | HUMMUS (¼ cup) | TUNA, IN WATER (½ can) |

Make the ultimate Pickle

Leave the feeble yellowed variety on the supermarket shelf and brine your own quick pickles for more delicious snacking. If you're craving something salty, chow on these instead of reaching for the chip bag for a (much) lower calorie option. These recipes come from Rick's Picks in Brooklyn.

BASIC QUICK DILL PICKLES

Good for burgers and sandwiches.

8   Kirby (pickling) cucumbers

1½   cups distilled white vinegar

3   cloves garlic, peeled and smashed

1   tablespoon kosher salt

1½   tablespoons sugar

1½   tablespoons pickling spice (available at grocery stores)

15   black peppercorns

5   sprigs dill

Slice the cucumbers lengthwise into four spears apiece and pack them into a 1-quart jar. In a medium pot, bring the vinegar, garlic, salt, sugar, pickling spice, and peppercorns to a boil over medium heat. Pour this hot pickle brine over the spears in the jar and stir in the dill sprigs. Let the pickles cool to room temperature, seal the jar, and refrigerate overnight to help develop the flavors. They'll last about 2 weeks in the fridge

MAKES 16 SERVINGS · PER SERVING 18 CALORIES // 0 G FAT // 362 MG SODIUM // 4 G CARBOHYDRATES // 1 G DIETARY FIBER // 1 G PROTEIN

FOR FLAVOR VARIATIONS, SKIP THE DILL AND TRY ONE OF THE FOLLOWING VARIATIONS.

MEXICAN QUICK PICKLES

Good for tacos.

2   teaspoons cumin seeds

2–3 jalapeño chile peppers, sliced thinly

1   red onion, sliced thinly

1   teaspoon kosher salt

KOREAN QUICK PICKLES

Good for Korean BBQ and cold sesame noodles.

2–4 teaspoons red-pepper flakes

2   cloves garlic, minced (in addition to the whole cloves already in the recipe)

2   scallions, sliced thinly

2   teaspoons sugar

1   tablespoon sesame seeds, toasted (to sprinkle on before serving)

SMOOTHIE SELECTOR

Not all snacks require chewing. In the universe of in-between meals, smoothies hold their own, especially when made with satiating, muscle-building whey protein. Whether you prefer to suck down your breakfast in liquid form or need a muscle-building protein boost before or after your workout, we've got all the smoothies you need right here. For every recipe, simply combine all the ingredients in a blender (preferably a heavy-duty one), pulse a few times, then run until smooth.

THE GREEN MONSTER

Fruit meets kale in this nutritional powerhouse. Try it, you'll like it.

1 scoop whey protein powder

½ cup plain yogurt

½ cup 2% milk or nut milk

1½ cups total strawberries and bananas

1 cup kale, ribs removed, roughly chopped

¼ cup ice

MAKES 1 SERVING · PER SERVING 395 CALORIES // 6 G FAT //
198 MG SODIUM // 57 G CARBOHYDRATES // 7 G DIETARY FIBER // 32 G PROTEIN

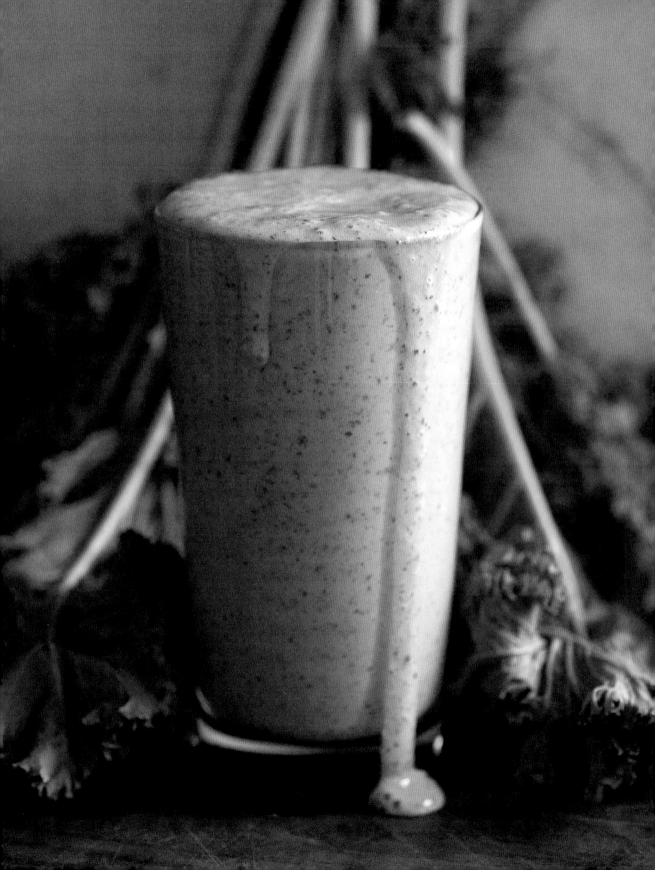

SMOOTHIE SELECTOR

THE ORANGEMAN

1 cup 1% milk

½ cup frozen orange juice concentrate

2 tablespoons low-fat plain yogurt

1 banana

2 teaspoons whey protein powder

6 ice cubes

MAKES 2 SERVINGS · PER SERVING 230 CALORIES //
2 G FAT // 70 MG SODIUM // 48 G CARBOHYDRATES //
2 G DIETARY FIBER // 8 G PROTEIN

HONEY-NUT CHEERY OAT

¾ cup unflavored instant oatmeal, nuked in water

¼ cup 1% milk

1 tablespoon peanut butter

2 teaspoons whey protein powder

1 teaspoon honey

1 teaspoon ground flaxseed

6 ice cubes

MAKES 1 SERVING · PER SERVING 144 CALORIES //
6 G FAT // 99 MG SODIUM // 17 G CARBOHYDRATES //
2 G DIETARY FIBER // 7 G PROTEIN

REAL ALMOND JOY

½ cup low-fat plain yogurt

1 banana

1 tablespoon almond butter

¾ cup orange juice

Dash of ground cinnamon

MAKES 1 SERVING · PER SERVING 366 CALORIES //
12 G FAT // 159 MG SODIUM // 15 G CARBOHYDRATES //
4 G DIETARY FIBER // 11 G PROTEIN

CEREAL KILLER

½ cup All-Bran Extra Fiber cereal

1 cup 1% milk

½ cup blueberries

1 tablespoon honey

2 teaspoons whey protein powder

6 ice cubes

MAKES 2 SERVINGS · PER SERVING 136 CALORIES //
2 G FAT // 121 MG SODIUM // 30 G CARBOHYDRATES //
7 G DIETARY FIBER // 7 G PROTEIN

NUT & BERRY

1 cup 1% milk

1 banana

½ cup raspberries

½ cup fat-free frozen yogurt

1 tablespoon peanut butter

MAKES 1 SERVING · PER SERVING 420 CALORIES //
9 G FAT // 235 MG SODIUM // 71 G CARBOHYDRATES //
8 G DIETARY FIBER // 18 G PROTEIN

THE NEAPOLITAN

¾ cup 1% chocolate milk

½ cup low-fat vanilla yogurt

¾ cup sliced strawberries

1 teaspoon ground flaxseed

2 teaspoons vanilla whey protein powder

3 ice cubes

MAKES 2 SERVINGS · PER SERVING 146 CALORIES //
3 G FAT // 102 MG SODIUM // 24 G CARBOHYDRATES //
2 G DIETARY FIBER // 8 G PROTEIN

THE ALMOND HAMMER

½ cup 1% milk

½ cup low-fat vanilla yogurt

¼ cup sliced almonds

2 teaspoons chocolate whey protein powder

1 teaspoon honey

1 teaspoon ground flaxseed

6 ice cubes

MAKES 2 SERVINGS · PER SERVING **168** CALORIES //
8 G FAT // **73 MG** SODIUM // **17 G** CARBOHYDRATES //
2 G DIETARY FIBER // **9 G** PROTEIN

PEANUT BUTTER OATMEAL SMOOTHIE

1 cup 1% milk

2 tablespoons low-fat vanilla yogurt

¾ cup unflavored instant oatmeal, nuked in water

2 teaspoons peanut butter

2 teaspoons chocolate whey protein powder

6 ice cubes

MAKES 2 SERVINGS · PER SERVING **161** CALORIES //
5 G FAT // **138 MG** SODIUM // **20 G** CARBOHYDRATES //
2 G DIETARY FIBER // **10 G** PROTEIN

STRAWBERRY SMOOTHIE

½ cup low-fat vanilla yogurt

1 cup 1% milk

2 teaspoons peanut butter

1 cup frozen unsweetened strawberries

2 teaspoons whey protein powder

6 ice cubes

MAKES 2 SERVINGS · PER SERVING **167** CALORIES //
5 G FAT // **125 MG** SODIUM // **22 G** CARBOHYDRATES //
2 G DIETARY FIBER // **10 G** PROTEIN

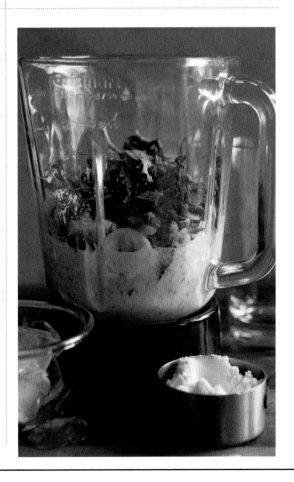

PB&J SMOOTHIE

¾ cup low-fat vanilla yogurt

¾ cup 1% milk

2 teaspoons peanut butter

1 banana

½ cup frozen unsweetened strawberries

2 teaspoons whey protein powder

4 ice cubes

MAKES 2 SERVINGS · PER SERVING **220** CALORIES //
5 G FAT // **131 MG** SODIUM // **35 G** CARBOHYDRATES //
3 G DIETARY FIBER // **11 G** PROTEIN

"UNHEALTHY" STUFF THAT'S ACTUALLY GOOD FOR YOU

Did you know there are more than 15 types of saturated fat? And despite the fact that they've been damned as a whole by nutrition experts for decades, some of them are actually heart healthy. That's good news, because high-fat foods are often the tastiest.

But a bad reputation is hard to shake. And though saturated fat is the most obvious example of a bad food gone good, it's not the only one. We've run the numbers and scoured the research to determine which vilified foods have been unjustly convicted. The result: six snacks and drinks that deserve an immediate pardon.

PORK RINDS

WHY YOU THINK THEY'RE BAD:
These puffy snacks are literally cut from pigskin. Then they're deep-fried.

WHY THEY'RE NOT:
A 1-ounce serving contains zero carbohydrates, 17 grams of protein, and 9 grams of fat. That's nine times the protein and less fat than you'll find in a serving of carb-packed potato chips. Even better, 43 percent of a pork rind's fat is unsaturated, and most of that is oleic acid—the same healthy fat found in olive oil. Another 13 percent of its fat content is stearic acid, a type of saturated fat that's considered harmless, because it doesn't raise cholesterol levels.

EAT THIS:
J&J Critters Microwave Pork Rinds
(microwaveporkrinds.com). Because the rinds are cooked and puffed in a microwave instead of deep-fried, each serving contains only 4 grams of fat—meaning they're lower in calories and less greasy than regular pork rinds.

ALCOHOL

WHY YOU THINK IT'S BAD:
It has little nutritional value and is the reason we need the term "beer belly."

WHY IT'S NOT:
In a study of more than 18,000 men, Harvard scientists discovered that those who had an average of two drinks every day, 5 to 7 days a week, had the lowest risk of heart attack. And researchers at the University of Buffalo found that men who consume that same daily amount have lower levels of abdominal fat than those who drink only once or twice every 2 weeks but down more than four drinks each time.

DRINK THIS:
Pinot noir. It contains more disease-fighting antioxidants than any other type of alcoholic beverage. Look for a Santa Barbara County pinot noir that's a 2002 to 2004 vintage; those are generally recognized as the top wine-producing years for this finicky grape.

BEEF JERKY

WHY YOU THINK IT'S BAD:
It's unhealthy meat that's loaded with preservatives.

WHY IT'S NOT:
Beef jerky is high in protein and doesn't raise your level of insulin—a hormone that signals your body to store fat. That makes it an ideal between-meals snack, especially when you're trying to lose weight. And while some beef-jerky brands are packed with high-sodium ingredients, such as MSG and sodium nitrate, chemical-free products are available. If you have high blood pressure, check the label for brands that are made from all-natural ingredients, which reduce the total sodium content.

EAT THIS:
Gourmet Natural Beef Jerky (available at americangrassfedbeef.com). It has no preservatives and is made from lean, grass-fed beef. Research shows that, unlike grain-fed products, grass-fed beef contains the same healthy omega-3 fats found in fish.

SOUR CREAM

WHY YOU THINK IT'S BAD:
You know 90 percent of its calories are derived from fat, at least half of which is saturated.

WHY IT'S NOT:
The percentage of fat is high, but the total amount isn't. Consider that a serving of sour cream is 2 tablespoons. That provides just 52 calories—half the amount that's in a single tablespoon of mayonnaise—and less saturated fat than you'd get from drinking a 12-ounce glass of 2% milk.

EAT THIS:
Full-fat sour cream. Unless you actually prefer the taste of light or fat-free products (and who does?), opt for the classic version; it tastes richer, and the fat will help keep you full longer.

COCONUT

WHY YOU THINK IT'S BAD:
Ounce for ounce, coconut contains more saturated fat than butter does. As a result, health experts have warned that it will clog your arteries.

WHY IT'S NOT:
Even though coconut is packed with saturated fat, it appears to have a beneficial effect on heart-disease risk factors. One reason: More than 50 percent of its saturated-fat content is lauric acid. A recent analysis of 60 studies published in the *American Journal of Clinical Nutrition* reports that even though lauric acid raises LDL (bad) cholesterol, it boosts HDL (good) cholesterol even more.

Overall, this means it decreases your risk of cardiovascular disease. The rest of the saturated fat is composed almost entirely of "medium-chain" fatty acids, which have little or no effect on cholesterol levels.

EAT THIS:
Shredded, unsweetened coconut. Have a handful as an anytime snack, straight from the bag. (Don't gorge; it's still high in calories.) It'll be filling, and it won't spike your blood sugar.

CHOCOLATE BARS

WHY YOU THINK THEY'RE BAD:
They're high in both sugar and fat.

WHY THEY'RE NOT:
Cocoa is rich in flavonoids—the same heart-healthy compounds found in red wine and green tea. Its most potent form is dark chocolate. In a recent study, Greek researchers found that consuming dark chocolate containing 100 mg of flavonoids relaxes your blood vessels, improving blood flow to your heart. What about the fat? It's mostly stearic and oleic acids.

EAT THIS:
Green & Black's Organic Dark 85%. The flavor is intense, but it'll help keep you from eating an entire bar. Just a square will do.

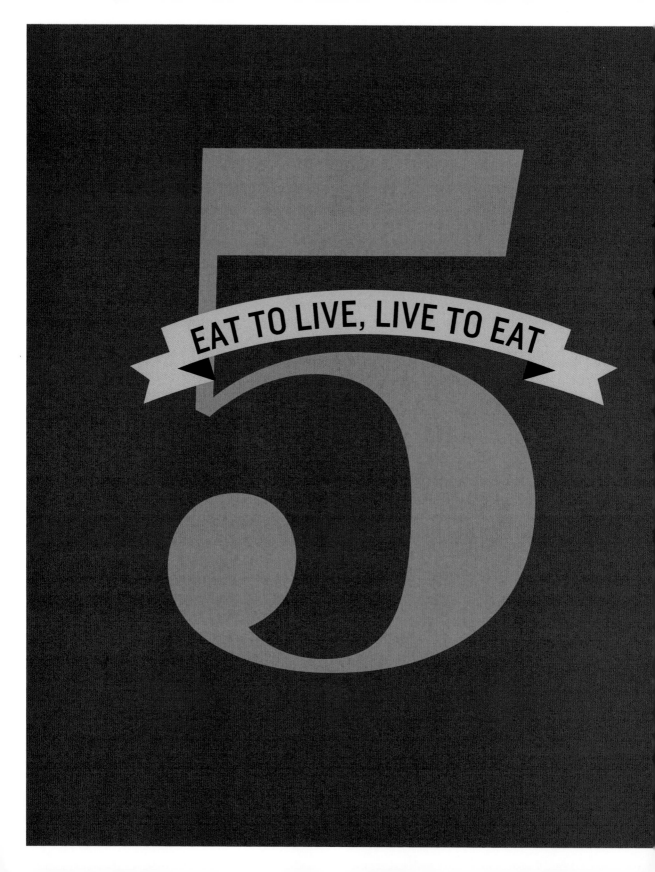

EAT TO LIVE, LIVE TO EAT

FAST WEEKNIGHT MEALS

When you come home tired and hungry, don't turn to a takeout menu. Just make one of these fast, protein-packed, delicious dinners.

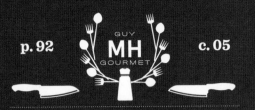

THE 5 RULES *for* COOKING ANY MEAL FASTER

You might think that cooking should be reserved for weekends, when you actually have the time (and energy) to fire up the stove. But with the right strategy, you can become a short-order cook in your own kitchen.

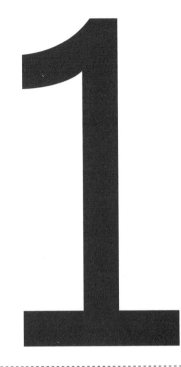

RULE N<u>o.</u>

1

SHOP ONCE, EAT FOR A WEEK

PLAN OUT WHAT you'll eat during the workweek. Shop on Sunday with one big list. Then you won't have to stop at the supermarket when the rest of the crowds hit it after work.

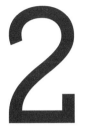

RUN A READ-THROUGH

IT SOUNDS OBVIOUS, but most guys don't do it: Before you even pick up an ingredient, give the recipe a good read. Not a scan. Not a skim. Read each step and work through it mentally in your head. You'll save yourself from screw-ups and surprises.

RULE N<u>o.</u>
3 | ## GATHER YOUR GEAR

PRIOR TO COOKING, pile up all the ingredients you need. Chefs call this "mise en place," which is a fancy term for having everything organized before you're ready to pull the recipe together. That way, you're not scrambling around the kitchen grabbing ingredients when you should be watching dinner cook.

RULE N<u>o.</u>
4 | ## SHARPEN UP

A DULL KNIFE can make slicing, dicing, and chopping more difficult—not to mention more dangerous. Learn how to sharpen your own knives on page 16. And place a damp kitchen towel or paper towel underneath you cutting board to prevent it from slipping when you cut.

RULE N<u>o.</u>
5 | ## HARNESS HEAT

IF THE RECIPE calls for a big pot of water or a hot pan, fire these up before you start working on your prep. For faster boiling water, add hot water to the pot, not cold, and use a lid. (And don't watch the pot!) If you're sautéing, heat your pans first and then add the fat.

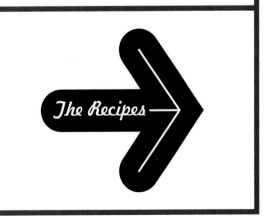

The Recipes →

CHILI-MANGO CHICKEN

Fresh mango tempers the spicy burn of the hot peppers in an Asian-inspired dish you won't find on the menu at your local Chinese restaurant. Serve this over brown rice.

1	pound boneless, skinless chicken thighs, cut into ½" pieces
1	tablespoon cornstarch
1	tablespoon lower sodium soy sauce
1½	teaspoons sesame oil
1½	teaspoons peanut or canola oil
1	red onion, chopped
1	tablespoon grated or minced fresh ginger
2	cups sugar snap peas
1	mango, chopped (see below)
1	tablespoon chili garlic sauce, preferably Huy Fong
	Ground black pepper

1. In a large bowl, combine the chicken, cornstarch, soy sauce, and sesame oil and let it sit for 10 minutes.

2. Heat the peanut or canola oil in a wok or large skillet over high heat. Add the onion and ginger and cook until the onion is translucent, 1 to 2 minutes. Add the peas and stir-fry for 1 minute. Add the chicken with its marinade and stir-fry until it begins to brown, about 2 minutes.

3. Add the mango, chili garlic sauce, and black pepper to taste. Stir-fry until the chicken is cooked through and the mango becomes saucy, about 1 minute more.

MAKES 4 SERVINGS · PER SERVING 355 CALORIES // 16 G FAT // 234 MG SODIUM // 19 G CARBOHYDRATES // 3 G DIETARY FIBER // 32 G PROTEIN

o DON'T MANGLE THE MANGO

STEP 1:
Set the mango on its narrow side. Start at the top, placing your knife about ½" from the center, and cut down to remove the fruit's wide sides. Then trim around the pit.

STEP 2:
Using a paring knife or the tip of a chef's knife, crosshatch the fruit's flesh, being careful not to slice through the skin.

STEP 3:
Push the skin inside out so the flesh protrudes in cubes. Then cut off the cubes.

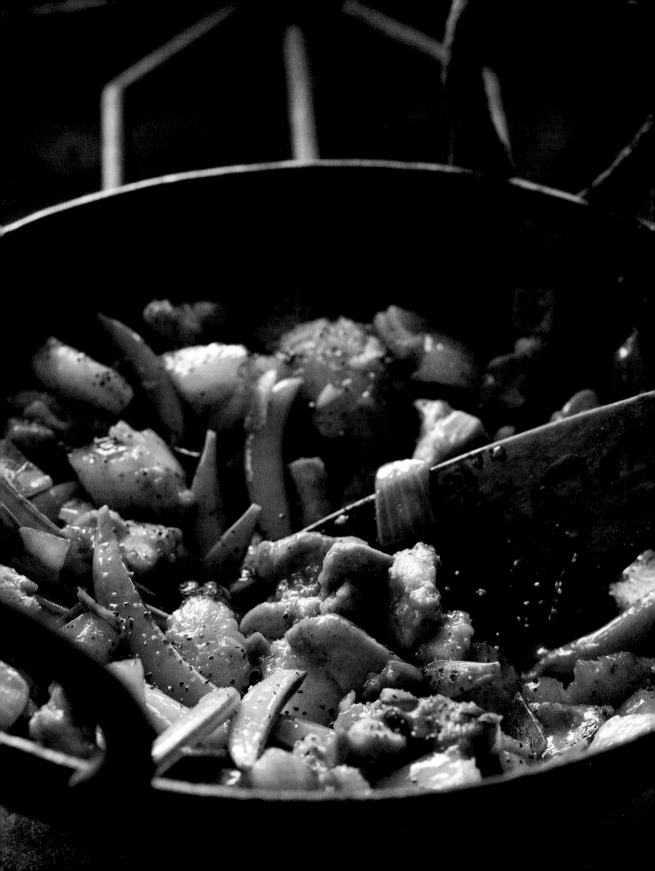

PERFECT STIR-FRY

"The key is having a few fresh vegetables, a lean protein, and a screaming hot wok," says Tyler Florence, the chef behind this recipe. He also recommends using a metal spatula to keep the meat and vegetables constantly moving, so everything cooks evenly.

1	tablespoon sesame oil
1	clove garlic, minced
1	tablespoon minced fresh ginger
4	ounces boneless, skinless chicken breast or pork tenderloin, sliced thin; or peeled and deveined shrimp
1½	cups bite-size pieces of vegetable (asparagus, mushrooms, peppers, broccoli, onions)
1	tablespoon lower-sodium soy sauce
1	tablespoon rice vinegar
1	tablespoon light brown sugar

1. Set a wok (or, failing that, a large stainless steel sauté pan) over high heat and coat the bottom with the oil.

2. When the oil begins to smoke, add the garlic and ginger and cook until lightly browned. Add the meat or shrimp and the vegetables and cook until the protein is cooked through and the vegetables have softened, about 8 minutes.

3. In a small bowl, mix the soy sauce, vinegar, and brown sugar. Add the soy sauce mixture (or a tablespoon of your favorite stir-fry sauce) to the pan and cook until everything is coated and the sauce has thickened, another 2 minutes. Serve by itself or with a scoop of brown rice and a hit of chili sauce. To change things up, keep different stir-fry sauces, like chili garlic and black bean, in the fridge.

MAKES 1 SERVING · PER SERVING 280 CALORIES // 7 G FAT // 628 MG SODIUM // 26 G CARBOHYDRATES // 4 G DIETARY FIBER // 30 G PROTEIN

SWEET-AND-SOUR PORK

Skip the sickly sweet takeout order and break out the wok to stir up this upgraded Chinese food menu staple.

---

2   tablespoons soy sauce

4   teaspoons rice wine or dry sherry

1   teaspoon sesame oil

¼   teaspoon coarse salt

¼   teaspoon ground black pepper

½   teaspoon + 2 tablespoons sugar

1   pound pork butt or shoulder, fat trimmed, cut into 1" cubes

½   cup all-purpose flour

½   cup + 1 tablespoon cornstarch

1   can (20 ounces) juice-packed pineapple chunks

⅓   cup ketchup

⅓   cup distilled white vinegar

1   cup + 1 tablespoon peanut oil or other vegetable oil

4   slices fresh ginger

1   green bell pepper, cut into 1" squares

1. In a large bowl, combine the soy sauce, rice wine or sherry, sesame oil, salt, pepper, and ½ teaspoon of the sugar. Add the pork, toss to coat, and marinate 10 minutes.

2. In another bowl, combine the flour and ½ cup of the cornstarch. Drain the pork, reserving the marinade. Lightly dredge the pork pieces in the flour-cornstarch mixture and set them aside on a plate.

3. Drain the pineapple chunks, reserving ½ cup of the juice. Add the juice to the bowl of reserved marinade and stir in the ketchup, vinegar, and remaining 2 tablespoons sugar and 1 tablespoon cornstarch.

4. Heat 1 cup of the oil in a 14" flat-bottomed wok until it's hot but not smoking. Add half the pork, spreading the pieces around in the oil. Cook 1 to 2 minutes until they begin to brown and then turn them. After 3 to 4 minutes, when the pieces are browned on all sides, transfer them to a plate lined with a paper towel. Repeat with the rest of the pork.

5. Rinse and dry the wok, and return it to high heat. Add the remaining 1 tablespoon oil and the ginger and stir-fry 10 seconds. Add the green pepper and stir-fry 1 minute. Add the reserved pineapple chunks and swirl the sweet-and-sour sauce into the wok. Bring the mixture to a boil, stirring until it's just thickened, about 1 minute. Add the pork and cook, stirring, for 2 to 3 minutes.

MAKES 4 SERVINGS · PER SERVING **498** CALORIES // **26 G** FAT // **721 MG** SODIUM // **40 G** CARBOHYDRATES // **2 G** DIETARY FIBER // **24 G** PROTEIN

SALMON TERIYAKI
with ASPARAGUS

This fast stir-fried meal makes cooking fish easy. Teamed with tender asparagus, you may have just found your new favorite way to chow down on omega-3s.

2	tablespoons lower sodium soy sauce
2	tablespoons mirin (sweetened rice wine)
1	tablespoon honey
1	tablespoon chili garlic sauce, such as Sriracha
1	teaspoon cornstarch
1	teaspoon sesame oil
1	tablespoon minced fresh ginger
2	cloves garlic, finely chopped
1	tablespoon vegetable oil, preferably peanut
1	pound skinless salmon (preferably wild), cut into 1" cubes
1	bunch asparagus, cut into thirds
	Cooked brown rice, for serving
1	tablespoon sesame seeds (optional)

1. In a small bowl, whisk together the soy sauce, mirin, honey, chili garlic sauce, cornstarch, sesame oil, ginger, and garlic. Set the mixture aside.

2. Heat a wok or large skillet over medium-high heat. When it's hot, add the vegetable oil and swirl to coat the pan. Add the salmon pieces and cook, stirring occasionally, until they just begin to turn opaque, about 2 minutes. Transfer them to a plate.

3. Add the asparagus to the wok and stir-fry until crisp-tender, about 2 minutes. Return the salmon to the wok and stir in the soy sauce mixture. Heat, stirring, for 1 minute. If the sauce seems too thick, add a couple of tablespoons of water. Serve over brown rice and garnish with sesame seeds.

MAKES 4 SERVINGS · PER SERVING **379** CALORIES // **12 G** FAT // **328 MG** SODIUM // **35 G** CARBOHYDRATES // **5 G** DIETARY FIBER // **31 G** PROTEIN

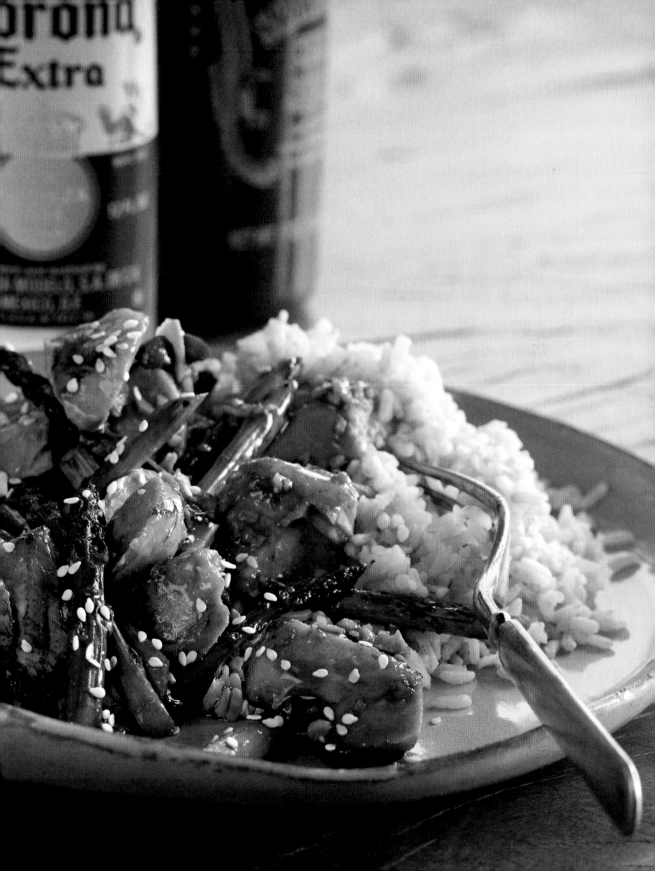

GENERAL TSO'S CHICKEN
with BROCCOLI

Admit it. It's the Chinese food dish you always wish you could order, but would regret having done so. This recipe dodges the deep-fryer, eases up on the sugary sauce, and even manages to sneak in some vegetables. Eat up—without the side of regret.

1	pound boneless, skinless chicken breasts, cut into 1" cubes
2	tablespoons + 2 teaspoons cornstarch
2	teaspoons vegetable oil, preferably peanut
2	cloves garlic, minced
1	tablespoon minced fresh ginger
¼	cup reduced-sodium chicken broth
1	tablespoon lower sodium soy sauce
1	tablespoon hoisin sauce
1	tablespoon rice vinegar
1	tablespoon honey
1	tablespoon chili garlic sauce, such as Sriracha
4	cups steamed broccoli florets, for serving
	Cooked brown rice, for serving

1. Preheat the oven to 375°F. Line a baking sheet with foil. On the baking sheet, toss the chicken chunks with 2 tablespoons of the cornstarch. Spread out the cubes and bake until they're cooked through, about 12 minutes.

2. Meanwhile, in a medium saucepan, combine the oil, garlic, and ginger and cook over medium heat, stirring often, for 2 minutes. Add the broth, soy sauce, hoisin, vinegar, honey, and chili garlic sauce and simmer 3 minutes. In a cup, whisk the remaining 2 teaspoons cornstarch into 2 tablespoons water. Add that to the pan and heat until the mixture has thickened, about 30 seconds.

3. Add the cooked chicken to the pan with the sauce and toss together. Serve alongside the broccoli and over brown rice.

MAKES 4 SERVINGS · PER SERVING **331** CALORIES // **7 G** FAT // **628 MG** SODIUM // **38 G** CARBOHYDRATES // **4 G** DIETARY FIBER // **30 G** PROTEIN

SKILLS

7 FAST WAYS TO EAT MORE VEGETABLES

Employ flavor enhancers strategically.

Forget limp, lifeless broccoli florets and sad, desiccated Brussels sprouts. Here are seven rapid-fire ways to make vegetables rival the meat they're paired with.

1

BRUSSELS SPROUTS

FLAVOR ENHANCER: Bacon
TECHNIQUE: Blanch halved Brussels sprouts in boiling water until crisp-tender. Drain. Crisp some chopped bacon in a skillet, add the sprouts, and cook until lightly browned. Season with salt, pepper, and fresh thyme, if you like.

2

BROCCOLI

FLAVOR ENHANCER: Brown butter and lemon
TECHNIQUE: Blanch broccoli in boiling water until crisp-tender. Drain. Heat butter in a large skillet, swirling until light brown. Add the broccoli and cook until it's lightly browned. Squeeze in lemon and top with toasted nuts.

3

SPINACH

FLAVOR ENHANCER: Nutmeg
TECHNIQUE: Combine 1 cup of cream with ¼ teaspoon nutmeg, 3 crushed garlic cloves, and salt and pepper, and simmer until reduced by half. Stir in 2 packages of thawed frozen spinach and heat through.

4

CARROTS

FLAVOR ENHANCER: Cumin seeds
TECHNIQUE: Gently boil ½ cup carrot slices in 1 cup each of water and orange juice, plus 1 garlic clove and ½ teaspoon cumin seeds, until the liquid has thickened enough to cling to the carrots. Finish with 1 tablespoon butter.

5

CAULIFLOWER

FLAVOR ENHANCER: Curry powder
TECHNIQUE: Break a head of cauliflower into florets. Toss with oil and then with 1 table-spoon curry powder. Roast in a 425°F oven until browned and tender.

6

GREEN BEANS

FLAVOR ENHANCER: Sofrito
TECHNIQUE: Sauté a chopped onion, 4 chopped tomatoes, and 2 minced garlic cloves in olive oil until very soft. Add 2 pounds green beans and simmer until just tender.

7

PEAS

FLAVOR ENHANCER: Prosciutto and mint
TECHNIQUE: Sauté 2 cups fresh or frozen peas in olive oil until barely tender. Fold in chopped fresh mint and thin strips of prosciutto.

ASIAN DUMPLING BOWL

In cooking, sometimes it's okay to take a shortcut. Attempt to make dumplings after work one night and you may not eat until early morning. Slide good-quality frozen dumplings into a flavorful broth, and you'll have a satisfying dinner on the table in mere minutes, says Iron Chef Masaharu Morimoto. A tip: If you don't have sake, just cook the dumplings according to package directions before adding them to the broth.

⅓	cup sake
20	frozen Asian dumplings (any variety)
5	cups low-sodium chicken broth
1	bunch bok choy, stalk ends trimmed
⅓	carrot
1	teaspoon sesame oil
½	bunch fresh cilantro, chopped

1. Heat the sake in a medium saucepan until simmering. Add a steamer insert and then the frozen dumplings, and cover. Steam until they're tender, about 10 minutes.

2. Bring the broth to a simmer in a large saucepan. Meanwhile, thinly slice the bok choy and carrot into 2" julienne strips.

3. Add the vegetables to the simmering broth and cook until crisp-tender. Add the steamed dumplings and cook 1 minute more. Serve the soup drizzled with sesame oil and garnished with cilantro.

MAKES 4 SERVINGS · PER SERVING **222** CALORIES // **9 G** FAT // **476 MG** SODIUM // **19 G** CARBOHYDRATES // **3 G** DIETARY FIBER // **16 G** PROTEIN

THAI BEEF LETTUCE WRAPS

Think of these wraps as an Asian play on tacos. Double the recipe to feed the family or a group of friends. Set the spread in the middle of the table, where everyone can personalize their wraps according to their tastes.

¾	pound flank, skirt, or sirloin steak
	Salt and ground black pepper
2	tablespoons fish sauce
	Juice of 1 lime, plus lime wedges for serving
1	tablespoon chili garlic sauce, such as Sriracha
1	jalapeño chile pepper, thinly sliced
½	red onion, thinly sliced
½	cup chopped fresh cilantro
1	carrot, grated
1	head Bibb lettuce, washed and dried, leaves separated

1. Preheat the grill or grill pan to high for at least 5 minutes. Season the steak with salt and black pepper and toss it on the grill. Cook for about 4 minutes on each side, until it's firm but yielding to the touch. Let it rest for 5 minutes.

2. In a small saucepan, combine the fish sauce, lime juice, and chili garlic sauce and heat over low heat.

3. Slice the steak thinly (if it's skirt or flank steak, be sure to cut across the grain) and drizzle half of the warm sauce over it. Set out the jalapeño and onion slices, cilantro, carrot, lettuce, lime wedges, and remaining sauce. Use the leaves like tortillas to wrap up the steak slices with the other ingredients.

MAKES 2 SERVINGS · PER SERVING **290** CALORIES // **8 G** FAT // **1,520 MG** SODIUM // **14 G** CARBOHYDRATES // **4 G** DIETARY FIBER // **40 G** PROTEIN

o JUICE CITRUS PROPERLY

First, heat it up. Cold citrus produces less juice. Either store your lemons, limes, and oranges at room temperature or zap them in the microwave until slightly warmed, about 15 seconds. Then, slice the citrus in half with a knife and plunge a fork into the flesh. Twist the fork as you squeeze the citrus half until tapped dry.

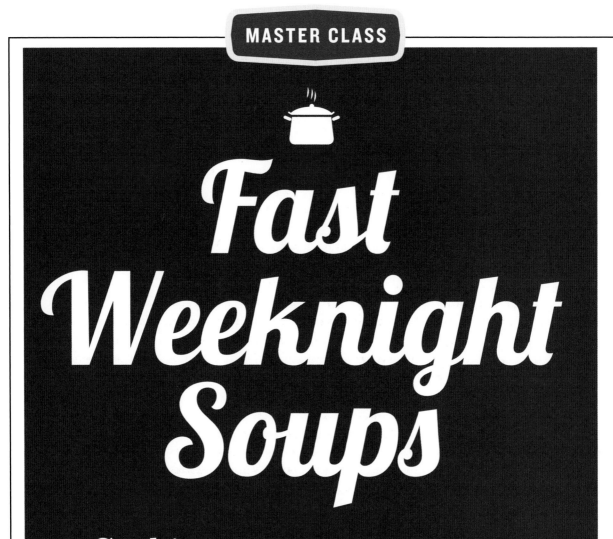

Fast Weeknight Soups

Cooking up a pot of soup doesn't mean you have to spend hours at the stove. Fact is, plenty of soups come together in mere minutes. Try one of these recipes alongside some seared steak, roast chicken, or stir-fried shrimp, and you'll see what we mean.

CREAMY CORN-POTATO CHOWDER

Heat 1 tablespoon of oil in a large saucepan over medium heat. Add 1 diced onion, 1 diced red bell pepper, and 2 minced cloves garlic and cook for 4 minutes. Toss in 2 cups frozen corn kernels, 1 pound diced Yukon Gold potatoes, 1½ cups low-sodium vegetable broth, 2 bay leaves, 1 tablespoon chopped rosemary, 1 teaspoon red-pepper flakes, 1 cup low-fat milk, and salt and pepper to taste. Bring to a boil and then reduce the heat and simmer, covered, until the potatoes are tender, about 15 minutes. Remove the bay leaves. Puree in the pot with a hand blender, or ladle half the soup into a blender, puree it, and return it to the pot.

MAKES 4 SERVINGS ·
PER SERVING **237** CALORIES //
5 G FAT // **129 MG** SODIUM //
44 G CARBOHYDRATES //
4 G DIETARY FIBER // **7 G** PROTEIN

CREAMY SPINACH-MUSHROOM SOUP

Heat 1 teaspoon olive oil in a large pot over medium heat. Cook 3 slices of bacon until crisp. Drain on paper towels. Remove all but 1 tablespoon bacon fat. Return to heat and add 8 ounces of sliced mushrooms. Cook about 5 minutes. Add 2 cleaned and sliced leeks and cook about 4 minutes. Stir in ½ cup dry white wine and simmer until reduced by half. Add a peeled and cubed russet potato and 5 cups water. Bring to a boil. Simmer about 15 minutes. Add 2 cups frozen peas and 8 ounces baby spinach and simmer 3 minutes. Puree the soup in a blender. Return to the pot and simmer. Add water if too thick. Remove from heat and stir in 2 tablespoons fresh lemon juice. Season to taste and ladle into bowls. Dollop with 2% plain Greek-style yogurt and sprinkle with reserved bacon.

MAKES 6 SERVINGS ·
PER SERVING **170** CALORIES //
4.5 G FAT // **222 MG** SODIUM //
23 G CARBOHYDRATES //
5 G DIETARY FIBER // **8 G** PROTEIN

BUTTERMILK PEA SOUP

Heat 1 tablespoon vegetable oil in a large saucepan over medium heat. Add 1 thinly sliced leek or onion and 2 minced cloves garlic and cook for 4 minutes. Stir in 4 cups reduced-sodium chicken broth, 3 cups frozen peas, 1 teaspoon ground cumin, 2 teaspoons dried thyme, ¼ cup fresh mint leaves, and salt and pepper to taste. Simmer for 15 minutes and then puree in the pot with a hand blender, or ladle into a blender and puree until smooth. Return to the pan, stir in ¾ cup buttermilk, and simmer 5 minutes more.

MAKES 4 SERVINGS ·
PER SERVING **194** CALORIES //
6 G FAT // **267 MG** SODIUM //
24 G CARBOHYDRATES //
6 G DIETARY FIBER // **13 G** PROTEIN

SPINACH SALAD *with* CORN, SHIITAKES, *and* BACON

Spinach salad with hot bacon dressing is delicious. We acknowledge that. But adding creamy bacon dressing to a salad is a good way to negate any nutritional value you pull from the greens. Instead, try this lighter version, made by Joe Yonan, author of *Serve Yourself*. Similar flavors, healthier dish.

1	tablespoon extra-virgin olive oil
1	slice bacon, cut into ½" pieces
4	ounces shiitake mushrooms, stems discarded, caps cut into ½" slices
1	cup corn kernels (fresh or frozen)
1–2	tablespoons sherry vinegar
	Kosher salt and ground black pepper
3	cups packed baby spinach

1. Heat the oil in a medium skillet over medium heat. When the oil starts to shimmer, add the bacon. Cook the bacon until crispy, 2 to 3 minutes. Use a slotted spoon to transfer it to a paper towel–lined plate.

2. Add the shiitakes to the pan and cook until they begin to sweat, 2 to 3 minutes. Add the corn and cook until it turns bright yellow, 2 to 3 minutes. Stir in 1 tablespoon of the vinegar. Taste and add more vinegar if desired. Season with salt and pepper.

3. Place the spinach in a serving bowl. Pour the hot mixture over the spinach and toss. Sprinkle the bacon pieces on top.

MAKES 1 SERVING · PER SERVING **431** CALORIES // **27 G** FAT // **557 MG** SODIUM // **45 G** CARBOHYDRATES // **9 G** DIETARY FIBER // **12 G** PROTEIN

SPICY BROCCOLI *with* SALAMI *and* FRIED EGG

The combination may sound strange, but give it a shot. Crushed red pepper flakes bring the heat to sautéed broccoli. The salami seasons the dish while boosting protein. And the fried egg? Break the yolk so its gooey deliciousness oozes over the entire dish.

---

1 cup broccoli florets

1 tablespoon olive oil, plus more for the eggs

2 cloves garlic, thinly sliced

¼ teaspoon red-pepper flakes

1 ounce salami, cut into thin strips

Salt and ground black pepper

3 eggs

1. Cook the broccoli in a large pot of boiling salted water until just tender, 3 to 4 minutes. Drain, rinse with cold water, and set aside.

2. Heat the olive oil in a cast-iron skillet over medium heat. Add the garlic and red-pepper flakes and cook, stirring, for 1 minute. Add the salami and broccoli and cook until the salami begins to brown. Season with salt and black pepper and keep warm.

3. In a separate skillet, fry the eggs sunny-side up in oil. Divide the salami and broccoli among 4 plates and top each with a fried egg.

MAKES 1 SERVING · PER SERVING **660** CALORIES // **39 G** FAT // **982 MG** SODIUM // **45 G** CARBOHYDRATES // **16 G** DIETARY FIBER // **43 G** PROTEIN

ITALIAN SEAFOOD STEW

This seafood stew couldn't be easier—and it'll see you through cold winter nights and back to grilling season.

1   tablespoon olive oil

1   bulb fennel, diced (reserve the fronds)

1   medium onion, diced

4   cloves garlic, roughly chopped

½   teaspoon fennel seeds

½   teaspoon red-pepper flakes

1   can (28 ounces) whole peeled tomatoes

12 ounces clam juice

1   cup chicken stock

1½ cups red wine (Pinot Noir)

2   bay leaves

½   teaspoon dried thyme

    Salt and freshly ground black pepper to taste

1   pound firm white fish, such as halibut or cod, cut into chunks

½   pound medium shrimp, peeled and deveined

12–16 mussels, scrubbed and debearded

1. Heat the oil in a large saucepan or pot over medium heat. Add the fennel, onion, garlic, fennel seeds, and red-pepper flakes and sauté until the vegetables are soft, about 5 minutes.

2. Lightly crush the tomatoes with your fingers (careful: juice may splatter from inside them) and discard the remaining tomato juice from the can. Add the tomatoes to the pan, along with the clam juice, chicken stock, wine, bay leaves, and thyme, and bring to a simmer. Cook for 5 minutes, taste, and adjust the seasoning with salt and black pepper.

3. Place the fish, shrimp, and mussels in the pan. Cook until the fish is firm, the shrimp are pink, and the mussels are open, about 5 minutes. Serve with the reserved fennel fronds for garnish.

MAKES 4 SERVINGS · PER SERVING 436 CALORIES // 10 G FAT // 1,000 MG SODIUM // 24 G CARBOHYDRATES // 5 G DIETARY FIBER // 48 G PROTEIN

QUICK CHICKEN ADOBO
and BLACK BEAN TACOS

Consider this recipe the fastest way to head south of the border. Stewed tomatoes serve as the base for a quick adobo-style sauce, and leftover rotisserie chicken cuts the cooking time way back. Add some black beans, jalapeños, and sour cream and you're eating *excelente*.

1	bunch cilantro, stems and leaves separated
1	can (14.5 ounces) no-salt-added stewed tomatoes
1	jalapeño chile pepper, halved and seeded
½	roasted chicken, skin and bones removed, shredded
	Salt and ground black pepper
1	can (15.5 ounces) low-sodium black beans, rinsed and drained
4	corn tortillas
¼	cup sour cream

1. In a blender or food processor, combine the cilantro stems, tomatoes, and jalapeño and puree. Transfer the mixture to a medium saucepan and bring to a boil over medium-high heat. Cook, stirring occasionally, until the sauce is thickened and reduced by half, 8 to 10 minutes.

2. Remove the sauce from the heat and stir in the chicken. Season with salt and black pepper to taste. Heat the beans in a small skillet over medium heat, stirring and smashing the beans with the back of a large spoon, until they're slightly thickened, 3 to 4 minutes. Season the beans with salt and black pepper.

3. Heat the tortillas in a dry skillet until warm and pliable. Assemble the tacos with the adobo chicken, beans, sour cream, and cilantro leaves.

MAKES 2 SERVINGS · PER SERVING **771** CALORIES // **21 G** FAT // **471 MG** SODIUM // **68 G** CARBOHYDRATES // **19 G** DIETARY FIBER // **73 G** PROTEIN

CHIPOTLE SHRIMP
with CILANTRO

Spicy chipotle peppers add smoky heat to this superfast seafood meal by chef Rick Bayless, master of authentic Mexican food. Serve it with a side of brown rice or use as a filling for warmed corn tortillas for a taco fix.

3	canned chipotle peppers in adobo sauce, plus 1 tablespoon of the sauce
1	can (15 ounces) diced fire-roasted tomatoes, drained
2	tablespoons extra-virgin olive oil
3	cloves garlic, finely chopped
	Salt
1	pound medium-large shrimp, peeled and deveined
¼	cup chopped fresh cilantro

1. In a blender or food processor, combine the chipotles, adobo sauce, and tomatoes and process until smooth.

2. Heat the oil in a large skillet over medium heat. Add the garlic and stir until fragrant and golden, about 1 minute. Pour in the chipotle-tomato mixture and cook, stirring frequently, for 5 minutes to meld the flavors.

3. Add enough water (about 1½ cups) to achieve a light tomato sauce consistency. Taste and season well with salt (about 1 teaspoon). Add the shrimp to the pan and cook, stirring, until the shrimp are opaque, about 4 minutes.

4. If the sauce seems too thick, stir in a little water. Serve the shrimp sprinkled with the cilantro.

MAKES 4 SERVINGS · PER SERVING **189** CALORIES // **9 G** FAT // **481 MG** SODIUM // **6 G** CARBOHYDRATES // **1 G** DIETARY FIBER // **21 G** PROTEIN

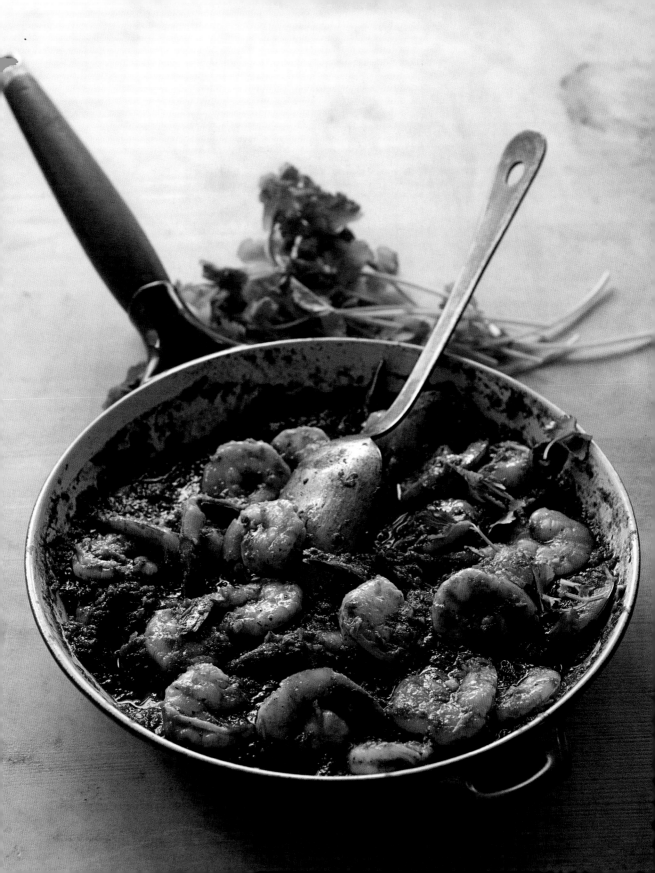

SMOKY *and* SPICY SAUSAGE HEROES

Sausage sandwiches can torpedo your gut with needless calories.
To adorn the lean sausage, this recipe swaps gobs of cheese for sautéed
peppers and onions, along with arugula for a peppery bite.

1	tablespoon extra-virgin olive oil
1	pound smoked turkey sausage
1	red bell pepper, thinly sliced
½	onion, thinly sliced
2	whole wheat sub or hero rolls (8-inch)
½	cup arugula
	Hot sauce

1. Heat the oil in a large, heavy skillet over medium heat until it shimmers. Add the sausage and cover the pan. Cook, turning the sausage links occasionally, until they're browned and cooked through, 10 to 12 minutes.

2. Remove the sausage from the pan and set aside. Add the pepper and onion and cook, stirring occasionally, until softened, about 8 minutes. Return the sausages to the pan and cook until hot, 1 to 2 minutes.

3. While the sausage is cooking, split and toast the rolls. When everything's ready, fill each roll with a piece of sausage and some pepper-onion mixture and arugula. Add hot sauce to taste.

MAKES 2 SERVINGS · PER SERVING **618** CALORIES // **26 G** FAT // **1,629 MG** SODIUM // **58 G** CARBOHYDRATES // **9 G** DIETARY FIBER // **41 G** PROTEIN

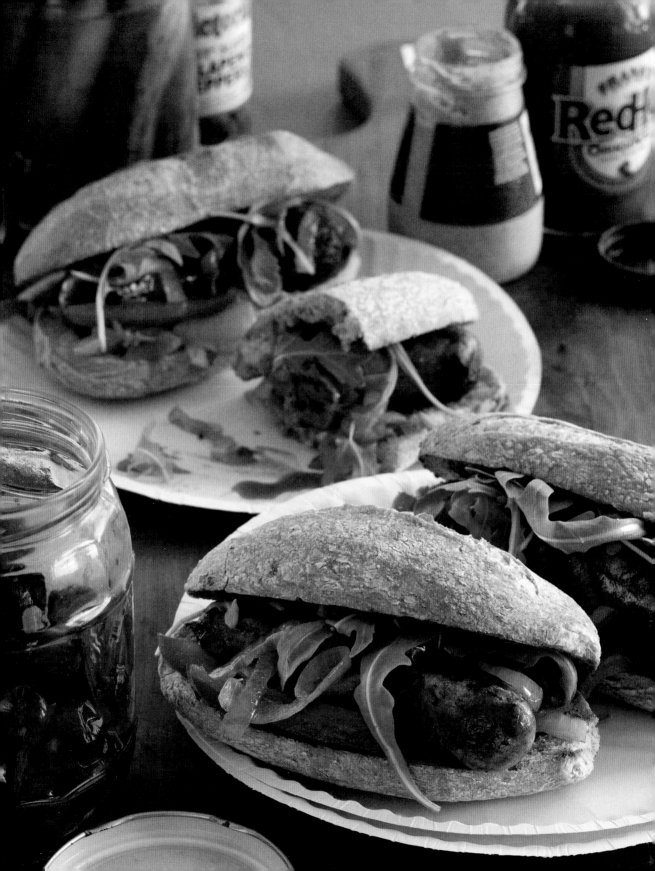

CHICKEN CACCIATORE

Adding dark to white chicken meat deepens the flavor of this all-in-one-pan dish, infusing the sauce with meaty flavor. It's so good you'll have it in heavy rotation for dinner options after your first bite.

2	tablespoons olive oil
8	boneless, skin-on chicken thighs (or a combination of thighs and drumsticks)
	Salt and ground black pepper
1	red bell pepper, thinly sliced
1	medium onion, thinly sliced
4	cloves garlic, minced
1	teaspoon red-pepper flakes
10–12	green or black olives, pitted and coarsely chopped
½	cup dry red wine
1½	cups chicken stock
1	pound Roma (plum) tomatoes, coarsely chopped
2	tablespoons chopped flat-leaf parsley

1. Heat the olive oil in a large sauté pan over high heat. Season the chicken with salt and black pepper to taste and add the pieces to the skillet, skin side down. Cook, turning occasionally, until they're deeply brown and crisp on all sides, 8 to 10 minutes. Remove them from the pan.

2. Reduce the heat. Add the bell pepper, onion, garlic, pepper flakes, and olives. Cook until the vegetables soften, about 10 minutes. Pour in the wine and simmer, stirring occasionally, until the wine nearly evaporates, about 5 minutes.

3. Add the stock, tomatoes, and chicken, tucking it skin side up into the vegetables. Bring to a simmer and cook over medium heat until the chicken is nearly falling off the bone and the sauce is reduced by half, another 20 minutes. Add salt and black pepper to taste. Sprinkle on the parsley.

MAKES 4 SERVINGS · PER SERVING **490** CALORIES // **29 G** FAT // **15 G** CARBOHYDRATES // **3 G** DIETARY FIBER // **360** MG SODIUM // **35 G** PROTEIN

PIT OLIVES FAST

You don't need a special widget to remove the pits from your olives. Just use a cutting board. Place the flat side of a chef's knife on each olive. Press down firmly. The olive's flesh will split, exposing the pit inside. Then pull the pit out. To save time chopping, pile up the pitted olives and use your chef's knife to rock through the pile until all the pieces are of similar size.

SHRIMP CREOLE

Cook up a taste of NOLA with this intensely flavored shrimp-and-vegetable dish by John Besh, executive chef of Restaurant August in New Orleans, Louisiana. Soul food, baby. The dish has a powerful garlic backbite and a foundation built from sautéed onion, celery, and green pepper (a classic Creole combination referred to as the holy trinity). Can't get your hands on fresh tomatoes? Sub in the canned variety.

4	tablespoons olive oil
2½	pounds jumbo shrimp, peeled and deveined
	Salt and ground black pepper
1½	medium onions, diced
½	green bell pepper, diced
½	rib celery, diced
5	cloves garlic, thinly sliced
2½	pounds tomatoes, chopped
1	bay leaf
1½	teaspoons red-pepper flakes
⅛	teaspoon ground allspice
	Sugar
	Cooked rice, for serving

1. Heat 2 tablespoons of the oil in a large, deep skillet over medium heat. Add the shrimp, season with salt, and cook until pink, about 2 minutes. Remove the shrimp from the skillet and set aside.

2. In the same skillet, heat the remaining 2 tablespoons oil over medium heat. Add the onions, bell pepper, celery, and garlic. Cook, stirring, until the vegetables begin to soften, about 2 minutes.

3. Add the tomatoes, bay leaf, pepper flakes, and allspice. Reduce the heat to medium-low, bring to a simmer, and cook for 10 minutes.

4. Return the shrimp to the pan and cook 1 to 2 minutes to meld the flavors. Season with salt, black pepper, and a little sugar (if the sauce tastes too tart). Remove the bay leaf. Serve the shrimp stew over rice.

MAKES 6 SERVINGS · PER SERVING **705** CALORIES // **20 G** FAT // **481 MG** SODIUM // **65 G** CARBOHYDRATES // **6 G** DIETARY FIBER // **65 G** PROTEIN

HONEY-MUSTARD SALMON
with ROASTED ASPARAGUS

Salmon is one tough fish. Unlike white varieties of fish, it can stand up to potent condiments like mustard. The cooking method in this recipe—first searing the fish and then finishing it in the oven—is a smart way to cook any kind of fish.

1	pound asparagus
2	tablespoons olive oil
¼	cup freshly grated Parmesan cheese
	Salt and ground black pepper
1	tablespoon unsalted butter
1	tablespoon light brown sugar
2	tablespoons Dijon mustard
1	tablespoon lower sodium soy sauce
1	tablespoon honey
4	salmon fillets (6 ounces each)

1. Preheat the oven to 400°F.

2. Toss the asparagus with 1 tablespoon of the oil, the Parmesan, and salt and pepper to taste. Place the spears in a baking dish and roast until they're crisp-tender, 10 to 12 minutes. (Leave the oven on for the salmon.)

3. Meanwhile, in a small microwaveable bowl, combine the butter and brown sugar. Microwave until they have melted together, about 30 seconds. Stir in the mustard, soy sauce, and honey.

4. Heat the remaining 1 tablespoon oil in an ovenproof skillet over high heat. Season the salmon fillets with salt and pepper, then add to the pan, flesh side down. Cook until browned on one side, 3 to 4 minutes. Flip the fillets, brush on half the honey mustard, and place the pan in the oven. Bake until the fish is firm and flakes easily (but before white solids begin to form on the surface), about 5 minutes. Remove the salmon from the oven and brush with more honey mustard. Serve with the asparagus.

MAKES 4 SERVINGS · PER SERVING **361** CALORIES // **17 G** FAT // **546 MG** SODIUM // **13 G** CARBOHYDRATES // **3 G** DIETARY FIBER // **39 G** PROTEIN

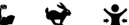

BLACKENED TILAPIA
with GARLIC-LIME BUTTER

The right seasoning can elevate inexpensive fish to restaurant-worthy
fare. Case in point: The blackening seasoning in this dish shotguns the
tilapia with a blast of heat while the acid of the lime juice brings
out the freshness of the fish.

1	lime
2	tablespoons butter, at room temperature
2	tablespoons chopped fresh cilantro
2	cloves garlic, finely minced
1	tablespoon canola oil
4	tilapia or catfish fillets
1	tablespoon blackening seasoning

1. Grate 1 tablespoon of zest from the lime into a small bowl. Then halve the lime and squeeze the juice (from both halves) into the bowl. Add the butter, cilantro, and garlic. Stir to blend and set aside.

2. Heat the oil in a large cast-iron skillet or sauté pan over high heat. Rub the fish all over with the blackening seasoning. When the oil in the pan starts to lightly smoke, add the fish and cook undisturbed until the spice rub becomes dark and crusty, 3 to 4 minutes. Flip and cook until the fillets flake with gentle pressure from your finger, 1 to 2 minutes more.

3. Transfer the fish to 4 serving plates and immediately top each with a bit of the flavored butter.

MAKES 4 SERVINGS · PER SERVING **323** CALORIES // **15 G** FAT // **115 MG** SODIUM // **4 G** CARBOHYDRATES // **2 G** DIETARY FIBER // **45 G** PROTEIN

Fast Pasta

When hunger strikes, a hearty bowl of noodles can always set you right, says Mark Bittman, author of *How to Cook Everything: The Basics*. Pasta satisfies the soul, fills the belly, and hits the table in mere minutes. Plus, it's a great way to pack in your vegetables—especially if you flip the traditional ratio of noodles to sauce so the pasta's still integral to the meal, just not the focus. Whether the sauce highlights vegetables, cheese, seafood, or meat, it's almost invariably the best part of the dish anyway. Start with these recipes and you'll discover that you can shift the balance of almost any pasta dish in favor of sauce supremacy.

ZITI WITH ASPARAGUS, PROSCIUTTO, *and* EGG

A silky egg and cheese sauce meets fresh asparagus and savory ham in this superfast pasta.

Cut 1½ pounds asparagus into 2-inch pieces. Heat 1 tablespoon olive oil in a large pan; add the asparagus and 4 ounces chopped prosciutto. Sauté until the asparagus is tender-crisp. Beat 2 eggs in a large bowl with ¼ teaspoon each of salt and pepper, and stir in the asparagus and prosciutto. Cook 1 pound ziti; drain and immediately add to the bowl. Toss until the pasta is well coated, adding pasta water as needed. Serve with ¼ cup grated Parmesan.

MAKES 4 SERVINGS ·
PER SERVING **590** CALORIES //
13 G FAT // **1,018** MG SODIUM //
87 G CARBOHYDRATES //
4 G DIETARY FIBER // **30** G PROTEIN

SPAGHETTI *with* ROASTED RAGU

Who needs to simmer a meat sauce when you can just throw all the ingredients in a pan and turn on the oven?

Peel a large eggplant and cut it into ½-inch cubes. In a roasting pan, toss the eggplant with ½ pound ground beef, a chopped onion, 2 minced cloves garlic, and salt and pepper; spread it evenly in the pan and drizzle on some olive oil. Roast at 425°F, stirring occasionally, until browned, 30 to 40 minutes. Add one 14.5-ounce can chopped tomatoes, drained; 3 tablespoons tomato paste; ½ cup dry red wine; and 1 tablespoon each chopped fresh oregano and thyme (or 1 teaspoon dried). Continue roasting until the mixture is thick, 10 to 15 minutes. Toss 1 pound cooked spaghetti with the sauce and top with ¼ cup grated Parmesan.

MAKES 4 SERVINGS ·
PER SERVING **654** CALORIES //
12 G FAT // **359** MG SODIUM //
102 G CARBOHYDRATES //
9 G DIETARY FIBER // **28** G PROTEIN

SPAGHETTI *with* LIMA BEANS *and* GOAT CHEESE PESTO

Pesto turns satisfying when it's paired with buttery beans and tangy goat cheese.

In a food processor, puree 2½ cups basil leaves, ½ cup olive oil, 2 ounces goat cheese, 2 tablespoons chopped walnuts, and 1 clove garlic. Cook 1 pound spaghetti until it's almost al dente; add 2 cups frozen lima beans and cook until heated through. Drain the pasta and beans and toss with the pesto, adding salt, pepper, and pasta water as needed.

MAKES 4 SERVINGS ·
PER SERVING **850** CALORIES //
36 G FAT // **393** MG SODIUM //
106 G CARBOHYDRATES //
9 G DIETARY FIBER // **25** G PROTEIN

LINGUINE *with* CLAMS *and* CHERRY TOMATOES

Briny shellfish and quick-roasted tomatoes pair together brilliantly in this recipe by Frank Castronovo and Frank Falcinelli, owners of Frankies 457 Spuntino in Brooklyn.

Preheat the oven to 400°F. On a baking sheet, toss 1 box cherry tomatoes with 1 tablespoon olive oil; season with salt. Roast until slightly shriveled, about 20 minutes. Meanwhile, heat 2 tablespoons olive oil in a large skillet over medium heat with 2 tablespoons minced garlic. Cook, stirring, until golden, 2 to 3 minutes. Add a large pinch of red-pepper flakes and 12 littleneck clams, scrubbed; cover the pan and reduce the heat to medium-low. Cook, shaking the pan occasionally, until the clams open, about 5 minutes. Toss ½ pound cooked linguine with the clam mixture, roasted tomatoes, and plenty of chopped parsley.

MAKES 2 SERVINGS · PER SERVING **775** CALORIES // **6 G** FAT // **148 MG** SODIUM // **98 G** CARBOHYDRATES // **6 G** DIETARY FIBER // **29 G** PROTEIN

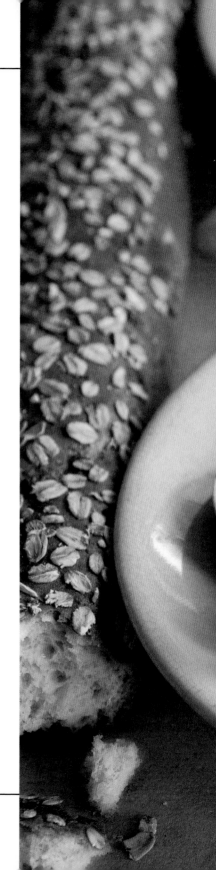

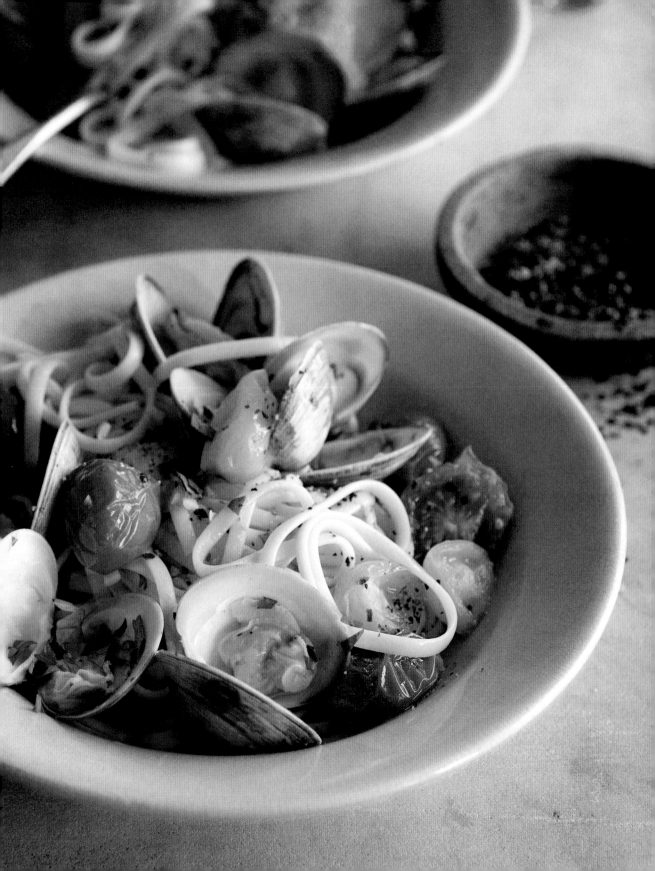

ZITI *with* CHICKEN, MUSHROOMS, *and* WALNUTS

Try this pasta from the late fall to late winter. The savory taste of the ingredients will fill your gut and warm your soul.

Heat 1 tablespoon olive oil in a skillet over medium heat and sauté 1 minced clove garlic until just fragrant, about 1 minute. Add ½ to ¾ pound sliced mushrooms and cook until their liquid releases and evaporates. Add ½ cup dry white wine and cook, stirring occasionally, until the wine reduces by half and the mushrooms begin to brown, about 5 minutes. Add 1½ to 2 cups shredded cooked dark meat chicken, season with salt and pepper, and cook until warmed through. Toss with 1 pound cooked ziti, ½ cup chopped walnuts, and lots of grated Parmesan.

MAKES 2 SERVINGS · PER SERVING **744** CALORIES // **38 G** FAT // **265 MG** SODIUM // **53 G** CARBOHYDRATES // **4 G** DIETARY FIBER // **42 G** PROTEIN

PASTA *with* EGGPLANT, LAMB, *and* PECORINO ROMANO

This Mediterranean-style pasta is bold and satisfying, thanks to plenty of earthy lamb.

Peel a large eggplant and cut it into ½-inch cubes. Heat 2 tablespoons olive oil in a large skillet on medium-high. Add the eggplant and cook until browned on all sides; drain on paper towels. Wipe the pan clean with a paper towel, return to medium heat, and add ½ pound ground lamb, a chopped onion, 1 minced clove garlic, and salt and pepper. Cook, stirring, until the meat is browned. Add ¼ pound cooked pasta, the eggplant, ½ cup grated Pecorino Romano, and ½ cup chopped fresh mint; toss with salt, pepper, and pasta water as needed.

MAKES 2 SERVINGS · PER SERVING **737** CALORIES // **43 G** FAT // **377 MG** SODIUM // **59 G** CARBOHYDRATES // **11 G** DIETARY FIBER // **30 G** PROTEIN

○ CLEAN UP YOUR OLIVE OIL BOTTLE

Block a slippery bottle: Wrap a (clean) sweatband around the top third of the bottle. That way, when you pour out the oil, the sweatband will absorb any oil dribbling down the side of the bottle.

BOIL PERFECT PASTA

Most people screw it up, says Marc Vetri, executive chef of Alla Spina
in Philadelphia. Allow Chef to school you.

1 GO DEEP

You want enough water in your cooking vessel to prevent the pasta from clumping together. So grab the largest pot in your kitchen (8- to 10-quart options work best for 1 pound of pasta) and fill it about three-fourths of the way full with hot water, to save time on boiling.

2 ADD SALT

Flip your burner's heat to high and salt the water heavily. If you're using an 8-quart pot, that's about 3 tablespoons of kosher salt. Most of the salt will stay in the water, leaving the pasta perfectly seasoned. Cover the pot with a lid to bring the water to a boil faster.

3 DROP AND STIR

When your water has reached a rolling boil, add the pasta and immediately stir. This will ensure the pasta does not stick together. There's no need to add olive oil—that doesn't help with sticking. Just continue to stir occasionally throughout the cooking process, leaving the lid slightly ajar when you're not stirring to encourage a rolling boil.

4 TEST WITH YOUR TEETH

Your goal is al dente—pasta that's just tender but still has a bite. Boxed pasta usually reaches al dente about a minute before the package instructions say to drain it. The only true way to check: Pull out a piece of pasta and bite into it.

5 FINISH IT

Pasta should never wait in the sink in a colander or else it will turn gummy. For a fast finish, set up your colander in the sink while the pasta cooks and have your sauce ready and waiting for the pasta. Reserve ¼ cup of the pasta water and drain the pasta. Then, return the drained pasta back to the pot, add the reserved pasta water, and then add the pasta sauce. The starches in the pasta water help the sauce cling to the pasta, creating a creamier, more flavorful pasta dish. Stir before serving.

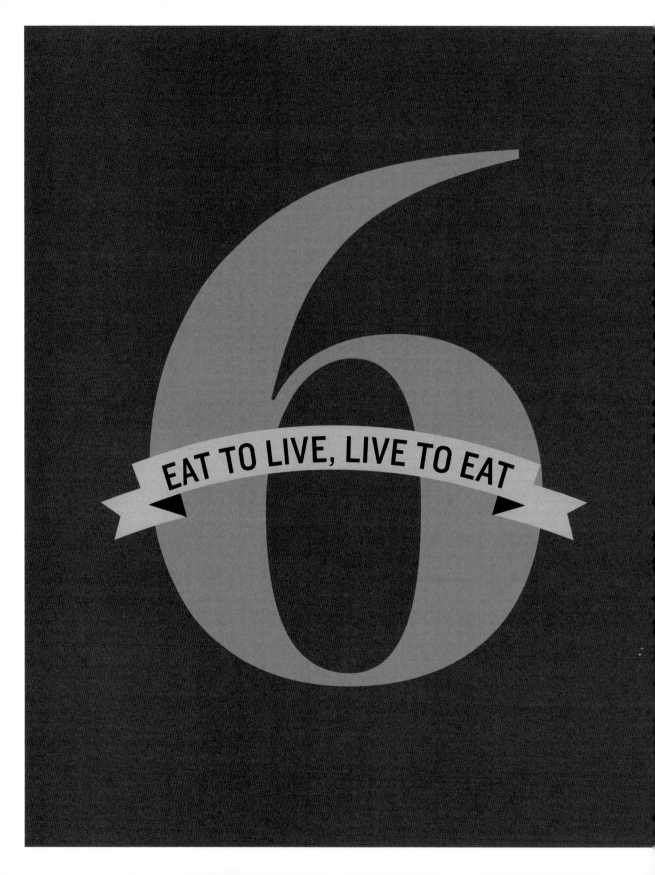

6

EAT TO LIVE, LIVE TO EAT

COOKING FOR A CROWD

Round up the crew.
These big-batch meals are
designed to feed the masses.

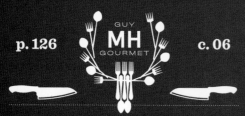

p. 126   c. 06

THE RULES *of* FEEDING FRIENDS

The recipes in this chapter have one single purpose: to help you cook great food for a large number of people with minimal hassle. But there are some principles you need to get down before you call everyone over.

1

DO THE MATH

IN THE RECIPES that follow, we've laid out the serving size for you, but there's a simple trick to calculating how much food you'll need to serve people at a party. Most eaters will consume 1/4 pound of protein per sitting. So whether you're buying shrimp, steaks—whatever—multiply 1/4 pound by the number of mouths you're feeding. Adjust the formula accordingly for friends named Bottomless Bob.

RULE N⁰. 2 | BANK ON THE ADVANCE

THERE'S NO NEED to wake up at dawn before a tailgate to prep a batch of chili. Block out the night before to cook your food and you'll save time and stress the day of the event. Plus, most big-batch meals actually taste better when they've overnighted in your fridge and had the time for the flavors to meld.

RULE N⁰. 3 | ARRANGE FOR TRANSPORT

SAVE THE FANCY dishes for Grandma and take the easy route when carrying your cooked food to its destination. Slow cookers and stockpots are durable enough to bang around in the back of your car on the way to the tailgate (just secure their lids with a few large rubber bands). Disposable foil roasting pans, like the kind you'd use for a Thanksgiving turkey, also work well, covered with aluminum foil, for hauling a large amount of wings. Plus, you can dispose of them on site after serving them up.

RULE N⁰. 4 | NAIL THE PRESENTATION

TOP CHEFS KNOW that the more mouthwatering their food looks on the plate, the more people will eat up with gusto. You don't have to go all Martha Stewart with this. Just use a large white plate to serve your food. For a simple way to garnish, take a few ingredients you used in the dish (herbs, citrus zest, grated cheese) and toss some more on top. No carrots carved like swans needed.

RULE N⁰. 5

DON'T FORGET

SERVING UTENSILS. How many times have we prepped a great meal for a crowd only to forget something with which to shovel it out of the pot? Don't forget the ladles and large serving spoons and forks. A tablespoon won't cut it. Also, don't forget the beer. Almost anything you cook will be appreciated all the more with a case of good beer on ice.

The Recipes →

NEW ORLEANS JAMBALAYA

New Orleans's answer to chili, jambalaya simmers several proteins with vegetables and spices into one big pot of chow that's worthy of gathering a crowd to eat well. We like this recipe from New Orleans chef John Besh.

1½	pounds andouille sausage, diced
1	pound fresh pork sausage, casings removed
1	pound bacon, diced
4	chicken legs, separated into thighs and drumsticks
	Salt and ground black pepper
5	ribs celery, diced
3	large onions, diced
2	green bell peppers, diced
6	cloves garlic, minced
1	tablespoon + 1½ teaspoons paprika
1	tablespoon cayenne pepper
1	teaspoon dried thyme
1	bay leaf
4½	cups converted Louisiana white rice
3	cups canned crushed tomatoes
3	cups rich chicken broth
2½	pounds shrimp, peeled and deveined
1½	pounds Louisiana crawfish, peeled and deveined (optional)
2	bunches scallions, chopped
1½	teaspoons celery salt

1. Preheat a large cast-iron pot over high heat. Reduce the heat to medium-high and add the sausages and bacon. Cook the meat as evenly as possible, stirring slowly, until the fat is released.

2. Season the chicken with salt and black pepper, add it to the pot, and increase the heat to high. Once the chicken has browned, add the celery, onions, bell pepper, and garlic. Continue to stir, allowing the ingredients to brown without burning.

3. Reduce the heat to medium and stir in the paprika, cayenne, thyme, bay leaf, and rice. Keep stirring for 5 to 7 minutes over medium heat.

4. Add the tomatoes and broth, increase the heat to high and bring to a boil, then cover and reduce to a low simmer and cook for 15 minutes.

5. Season the shrimp and crawfish (if using) with salt and pepper, and add them to the pot. Keep the pot covered for an additional 5 minutes before removing from the heat and adding the scallions. Check for seasonings. Add the celery salt and salt and pepper to taste.

MAKES 16 SERVINGS · PER SERVING **648** CALORIES // **31 G** FAT // **1,233 MG** SODIUM // **53 G** CARBOHYDRATES // **3 G** DIETARY FIBER // **38 G** PROTEIN

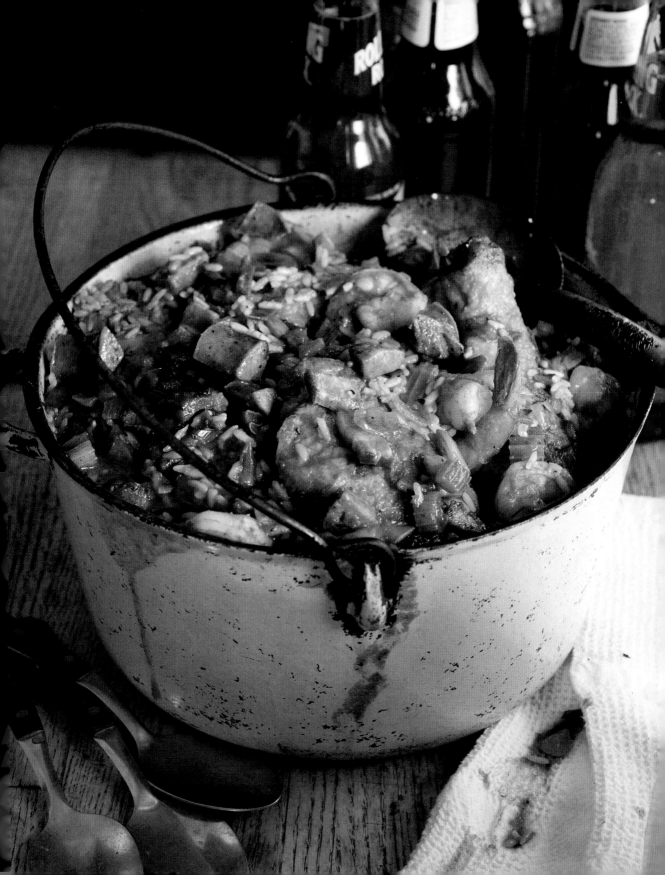

SPICY MONTEREY JACK *and* CHEDDAR GRILLED CHEESE

You've never had a grilled cheese like this one. It's constructed by Thomas Keller, world-famous chef of The French Laundry in Napa Valley, California. Gooey, spicy, and rich, this upgraded childhood favorite is a great way to feed the fans at game night. Just bump up the ingredient amounts according to how many people are coming over.

1 or 2 jalapeño chile peppers

1   red bell pepper

    Butter, at room temperature

4   slices brioche, whole wheat, or sourdough bread (¾" thick)

4   slices Monterey Jack cheese

4   slices cheddar cheese

1. Fill a bowl with ice water. Place the jalapeños and bell pepper on a baking sheet and fire up a small butane torch (we like the Weller Table Top butane torch, sears.com) until the flame burns blue. Carefully blister the skins of the peppers with the blowtorch, turning them with a fork as you work.

2. Pull on a pair of plastic gloves and plunge the peppers into the ice water for a few seconds. Then rub off their skins, halve lengthwise, seed, and chop.

3. Preheat a cast-iron skillet over medium heat. For each sandwich, liberally butter both sides of two bread slices. Place 2 slices of Monterey Jack on one piece of bread; add a heaping tablespoon of the pepper mixture in the middle. Place 2 slices of cheddar on the other piece of bread, and put the bread slices together.

4. Place the sandwiches in the skillet over medium heat, and cook until the bread is golden brown and the cheeses melt together, 3 to 5 minutes a side. Cut them in half diagonally and serve with beer.

MAKES 2 SERVINGS · PER SERVING **681** CALORIES // **46 G** FAT // **1,028 MG** SODIUM // **35 G** CARBOHYDRATES // **5 G** DIETARY FIBER // **34 G** PROTEIN

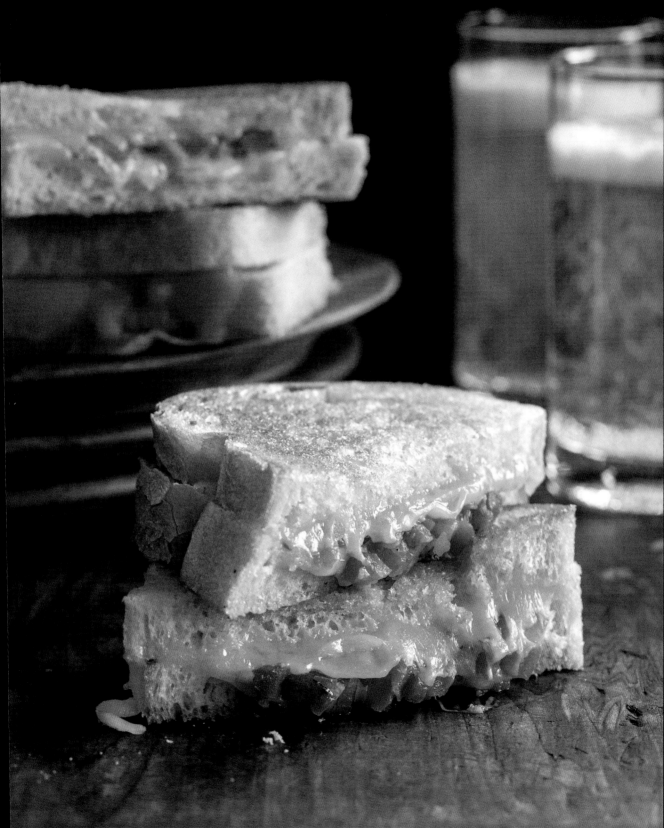

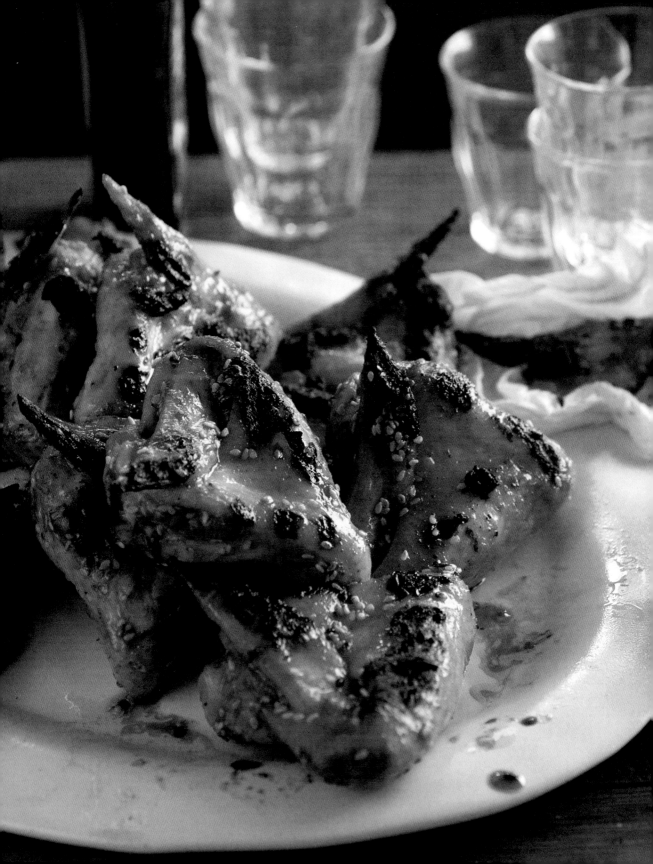

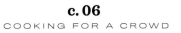

WING NIGHT

Chicken wings aren't

always bad for you. It's when the cook at your local bar batters them, dunks them into a greasy fryer, and pushes them out in buckets that the bird goes bust. Your can still enjoy the fire and flavor of wing night by nixing the deep fryer. Grilled or baked wings are better for you because those healthier cooking styles drain some of the calorie-laden fat. The marinade is what delivers the punch to your taste buds. Try these recipes from top-seeded chefs.

Gochujang pepper paste gives these Korean BBQ wings crazy heat and depth. PAGE 135

WING NIGHT

WING IT

1 PREP THE CHICKEN

Rinse 2 to 4 pounds of whole wings and pat dry.
This is enough to serve 4 to 6 people.

2 MARINATE THE WINGS*

Combine the flavorings in a bowl or resealable plastic bag and add the wings.
Follow the instructions for the proper marinade times—
it's crucial to developing flavors.

3 BAKE

Preheat the oven to 400°F. Line a baking sheet with foil, brush it with
olive oil, and spread the wings out on it. Bake the wings for 20 minutes,
turn them, and bake until the meat is no longer pink, about
20 more minutes.

(OR)

3 GRILL

Preheat a grill to medium-low. Cook the wings, covered, over
indirect heat for 10 to 15 minutes on each side, or until they bounce after
you drop them from 6 inches above the grill.

*Pepper Sergeants: Don't blame us for scorched tastebuds: The hot wing marinade recipes
on the following pages are courtesy of Jet Tila, executive chef of The Charleston in
Santa Monica (Korean BBQ); Shawn McClain, chef and owner of Green Zebra in Chicago (Chili Garlic);
and Elizabeth Karmel, executive chef of Hill Country, New York City (Inferno).

KOREAN BBQ WINGS

MAKE THE MARINADE:

½ cup soy sauce

⅓ cup light brown sugar

⅓ cup Korean pepper paste (optional)

2 tablespoons sesame oil

3 or 4 cloves garlic

3 or 4 scallions, chopped

2 to 3 tablespoons toasted sesame seeds

Salt and ground black pepper to taste

MARINATE THE WINGS:

At least 4 hours or up to overnight

FINISH THE WINGS:

Top the cooked wings with more chopped scallions and a shake of sesame seeds

MAKES 4 SERVINGS ·

PER SERVING **464** CALORIES // **32 G** FAT // **948 MG** SODIUM // **7 G** CARBOHYDRATES // **0 G** DIETARY FIBER // **35 G** PROTEIN

LIGHTENED-UP BUFFALO WINGS

MAKE THE MARINADE:

1 cup Frank's RedHot

¼ teaspoon ground red pepper

MARINATE THE WINGS:

30 minutes, up to 4 hours

MAKE THE SAUCE:

In a medium bowl, combine:

1 cup 2% Greek yogurt

1 teaspoon garlic powder

1 teaspoon ground black pepper

½ cup blue cheese

A few dashes Worcestershire sauce

2 tablespoons white wine vinegar

FINISH THE WINGS:

Serve the wings with the blue cheese sauce and celery sticks.

MAKES 6 SERVINGS ·

PER SERVING **436** CALORIES // **29 G** FAT // **1,761 MG** SODIUM // **9 G** CARBOHYDRATES // **3 G** DIETARY FIBER // **35 G** PROTEIN

○ TOAST SESAME SEEDS RIGHT

Unless you find a jar of toasted sesame seeds in the Asian section of your supermarket, you'll want to toast your own to bring out that nutty flavor. Place the seeds in a medium dry skillet and set over medium heat. Toast, stirring the seeds frequently, until they turn golden, 3 to 5 minutes.

WING NIGHT

CHILI-GARLIC WINGS

MAKE THE MARINADE:

1 cup Thai sweet chili sauce

1 tablespoon chili garlic sauce, such as Sriracha

2 tablespoons fish sauce

1 teaspoon minced garlic

2 tablespoons finely chopped cilantro, plus more for serving

MARINATE THE WINGS:

Reserve ¼ cup marinade for dipping; marinate wings for 2 hours

FINISH THE WINGS:

Top the cooked wings with more cilantro

MAKES 4 SERVINGS ·
PER SERVING **476** CALORIES // **29 G** FAT //
789 MG SODIUM // **13 G** CARBOHYDRATES //
0 G DIETARY FIBER // **34 G** PROTEIN

INFERNO WINGS

MAKE THE RUB:

2 teaspoons each
black pepper, white pepper,
garlic powder, onion powder,
sweet Spanish paprika, dry mustard,
dried oregano, dried sage,
dried rosemary

MAKE THE SAUCE:

¼ cup each
jalapeño hot sauce, Louisiana hot sauce, Tabasco sauce, barbecue sauce

3 tablespoons each
Worchestershire sauce, liquid from jar of jalapeños (see below)

3 tablespoons cayenne pepper

3 tablespoons red-pepper flakes

3 pickled jalapeño peppers,
cut into slices

MARINATE THE WINGS:

30 minutes rubbed with dry spices

FINISH THE WINGS:

Combine liquids, cayenne, chili flakes, and wings in a pan; cover and bake for 15 minutes, stirring often. Top with jalapeño slices.

MAKES 4 SERVINGS ·
PER SERVING **520** CALORIES // **32 G** FAT //
1,203 MG SODIUM // **20 G** CARBOHYDRATES //
5 G DIETARY FIBER // **37 G** PROTEIN

SIRLOIN STEAKS *with* BACON–BLUE CHEESE BUTTER

If you're going to have a few buddies over, go all out. This recipe from butcher Tom Mylan of the Meat Hook in Brooklyn, New York, starts with a slab of sirloin, which you then cut into superthick steaks. Bigger steaks require bolder flavors, so finish strong with a topping of cheese-infused butter. Over the top? A little. But we're sure your friends won't mind.

1   **stick (4 ounces) salted butter, at room temperature**

2   **tablespoons bacon fat (save from your last batch of bacon)**

2   **tablespoons crumbled blue cheese**

2   **tablespoons thinly sliced scallions**

    Salt and ground pepper

1   **top-sirloin roast (6 to 7 pounds), cut into steaks**

1. Preheat the oven to 375°F. In a bowl, combine the butter, bacon fat, cheese, and scallions. Season with salt and pepper. On a piece of plastic wrap, roll the mixture into a log. Put it in the freezer.

2. Season the steaks with salt and pepper. Heat two heavy ovenproof pans on high. (Open the windows and turn on your stove's fan.) When they're blazing hot, add one or two steaks to each pan; sear until a crust develops, 2 to 3 minutes on each side.

3. Transfer the pans to the oven and cook to medium-rare, 5 to 7 minutes. Slice the butter into ½"-thick rounds, place them on the steaks, and let the meat rest 5 minutes before serving.

MAKES 8 SERVINGS · PER SERVING **584** CALORIES // **29 G** FAT // **345 MG** SODIUM // **0 G** CARBOHYDRATES // **0 G** DIETARY FIBER // **76 G** PROTEIN

○ CUT YOUR OWN STEAKS

Supermarket steaks cook up dry because they're too thin. It's time to cut your own.

1   Place a roast on a cutting board and examine it for its striations—the "grain." Position it so the grain runs perpendicular to your knife. (If you cut parallel to the grain, your meal will turn out tough.)

2   Holding the roast in place, use a chef's knife to slice it into steaks 1½" to 2" thick; use long, even strokes, drawing the knife toward you. (Resist the urge to saw with the knife.)

Chili

You never know with bowl games.
It's 50-50 whether the college kids will produce
fourth-quarter heroics or second-quarter blowouts.
Not so with the traditional halftime meal, the
Chili Bowl. It reliably unites heat, spice, protein,
and fiber, with spectacular results.

ANCHO, BEEF, *and* BULGUR CHILI

Chili purists might argue the virtues of a beanless bowl, but the fiber in beans keeps you feeling satisfied and may also help regulate blood pressure and boost heart health. To ramp up the fiber even more, add bulgur, a type of cracked wheat that's a ground beef lookalike and adds even more meaty texture.

1	tablespoon + 1 teaspoon olive oil
1	large onion, coarsely chopped
1	green bell pepper, diced
1–2	serrano chiles, seeded and chopped
3	cloves garlic, thinly sliced
1½	teaspoons ground cumin
1	teaspoon ancho chile powder
¾	teaspoon dried oregano, crumbled
½	teaspoon ground cinnamon
⅓	cup bulgur wheat
1	pound 90% lean ground sirloin
1	can (15 ounces) whole tomatoes in puree
1	can (15 ounces) black beans, rinsed and drained
½	cup water
1	teaspoon coarse salt
	Lime wedges (optional)

1. In a 5-quart pot, heat the oil over medium heat. Add the onion, bell pepper, serranos, and garlic and cook, stirring occasionally, until the onion is golden brown and the peppers are tender, about 10 minutes.

2. Add the cumin, ancho powder, oregano, and cinnamon and cook, stirring, for 1 minute to lightly toast them. Stir in the bulgur. Add the beef and cook, breaking it up with a spoon, until it's no longer pink, about 3 minutes.

3. Stir in the tomatoes and their puree, the beans, water, and salt and bring to a simmer. Cover and cook until the flavors are blended and the meat and bulgur are tender, about 30 minutes. Serve with lime wedges if desired.

MAKES 4 SERVINGS · PER SERVING 317 CALORIES // 10 G FAT // 1,134 MG SODIUM // 31 G CARBOHYDRATES // 9 G DIETARY FIBER // 29 G PROTEIN

FOUR-ALARM GREEN CHILI *with* PORK

Along with your big pot and your wooden spoon, keep a fire extinguisher on hand when dealing with this recipe. With three varieties of hot peppers and chipotle chile powder, you're going to need more cooling power than a beer to help handle the heat.

1	pound tomatillos, husks removed
2	poblano peppers, halved lengthwise
2	serrano chile peppers, halved lengthwise
1	pickled jalapeño pepper, halved lengthwise
1	small onion, cut into chunks
3	cloves garlic, smashed and peeled
½	cup fresh cilantro
1	teaspoon dried oregano
1	teaspoon ground cumin
½	teaspoon chipotle chile powder
½	teaspoon ground coriander
¼	teaspoon ground allspice
¼	cup water
2	tablespoons olive oil
1½	pounds boneless pork shoulder (butt), cut into 1" chunks
1½	teaspoons coarse salt
1	tablespoon lime juice

1. Cook the tomatillos in a medium pot of boiling water until softened, about 5 minutes. Drain and transfer to a blender along with all the peppers, the onion, garlic, cilantro, and dried herbs and spices. Add the water and puree until smooth.

2. Meanwhile, in a 5-quart pot, heat the oil over medium-high heat. Season the pork with ½ teaspoon of the salt. Add half the pork to the pot and sear it until the chunks are browned, about 7 minutes. Transfer the pork to a bowl. Repeat with the remaining pork.

3. Add the tomatillo puree to the pot and cook for 3 minutes. Return the seared pork and add the lime juice and remaining 1 teaspoon salt. Bring to a boil, then reduce to a simmer, cover, and cook, stirring occasionally, until the pork is tender, about 1 hour 15 minutes.

MAKES 4 SERVINGS · PER SERVING **465** CALORIES // **31 G** FAT // **849 MG** SODIUM // **13 G** CARBOHYDRATES // **4 G** DIETARY FIBER // **13 G** PROTEIN

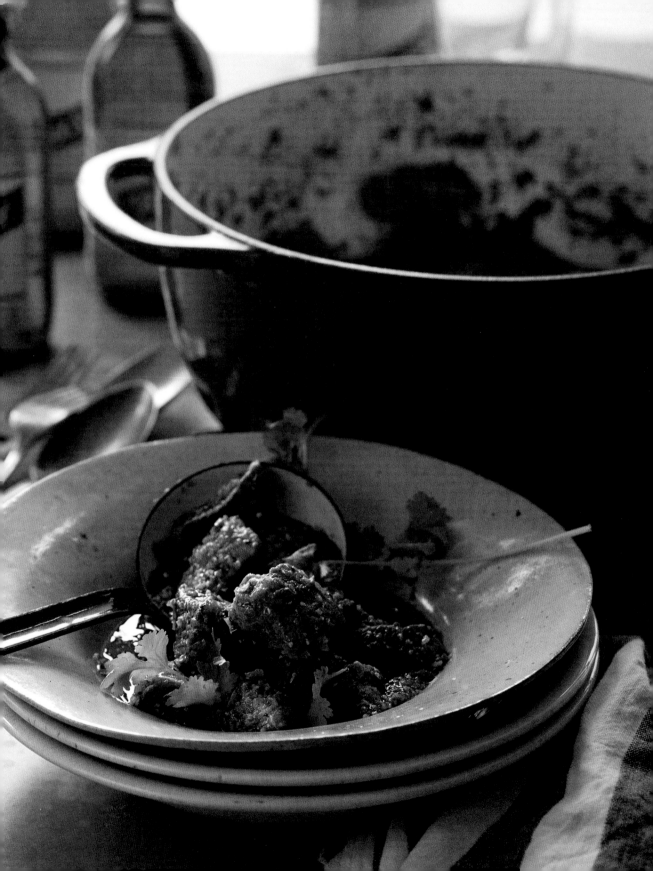

CHUNKY TEX-MEX CHILI

Like some NFL playoff teams, lean meats are overrated.
Zero-fat ground turkey breast has zero taste. If you want to cut calories
while still creating a championship bowl of Texas red, stick to
relatively lean cubed dark-meat chicken or beef sirloin. They both
turn tender and flavorful when slow-simmered.

4	teaspoons olive oil
1	small fresh chorizo sausage (3 ounces), casing removed (optional)
1¼	pounds boneless beef sirloin (choose the most marbled) or boneless, skinless chicken thighs, cut into ½" chunks
1	medium onion, coarsely chopped
3	cloves garlic, thinly sliced
¼	cup ancho chile powder
2	teaspoons dried oregano
¼	cup tomato paste
1	tablespoon red wine vinegar
1¼	cups water
1	teaspoon coarse salt
2	tablespoons cornmeal

1. In a 5-quart pot, heat 2 teaspoons of the oil over medium heat. Add the chorizo (if using) and cook until it has rendered its fat, about 5 minutes. Remove it to a bowl with a slotted spoon.

2. Add half the meat to the pot and cook until browned, about 5 minutes. Transfer with a slotted spoon to the bowl with the chorizo. Repeat with the remaining meat.

3. Add the onion, garlic, and remaining 2 teaspoons oil to the pot and cook, stirring frequently, until the onion is tender, about 7 minutes. Stir in the ancho powder and oregano, and cook 1 minute. Stir in the tomato paste and vinegar.

4. Return the meat and chorizo to the pot along with the water and salt, and bring to a boil. Reduce to a simmer, cover, and cook, stirring occasionally, until the meat is tender, about 1 hour. Stir in the cornmeal and simmer until lightly thickened, about 5 minutes.

MAKES 4 SERVINGS · PER SERVING 230 CALORIES // 9 G FAT // 850 MG SODIUM // 14 G CARBOHYDRATES // 4 G DIETARY FIBER // 24 G PROTEIN

WINTER-VEGETABLE CHILI

On paper, vegetarian chili sounds like a smart idea—the hidden-ball trick for your daily servings. The problem: All-veg varieties taste like ... vegetables! The solution: Choose produce that actually works with Mexican flavors, and don't skimp on fresh toppings like tomato, avocado, and pickled jalapeños.

2	tablespoons olive oil
1	large onion, coarsely chopped
3	cloves garlic, thinly sliced
1	red bell pepper, diced
2	cups finely chopped cabbage (you can use pre-shredded coleslaw mix)
1	tablespoon unsweetened cocoa powder
1	teaspoon chipotle chile powder
1	pound butternut squash, peeled and cut into 1" chunks (3 cups)
¼	cup tomato paste
2	cups vegetable broth
1	can (15 ounces) kidney beans, rinsed and drained
1	can (15 ounces) chickpeas, rinsed and drained
1½	teaspoons coarse salt
1½	cups frozen corn kernels, thawed
	Avocado, tomato, and pickled jalapeños, for topping

1. In a 5-quart pot, heat the oil over medium heat. Add the onion, garlic, and bell pepper and cook, stirring frequently, until the onion is golden brown and tender, about 10 minutes.

2. Stir in the cabbage and cook, stirring frequently, until it's wilted, about 5 minutes. Add the cocoa powder and chipotle powder and cook 1 minute. Add the squash and tomato paste and cook 1 minute.

3. Add the broth, beans, chickpeas, and salt and bring to a boil. Reduce to a simmer, cover, and cook until the squash is tender, about 30 minutes. Stir in the corn and heat through, about 3 minutes longer. Serve topped with avocado, tomato, and jalapeños.

MAKES 4 SERVINGS · PER SERVING 372 CALORIES // 9 G FAT // 1,644 MG SODIUM // 66 G CARBOHYDRATES // 14 G DIETARY FIBER // 13 G PROTEIN

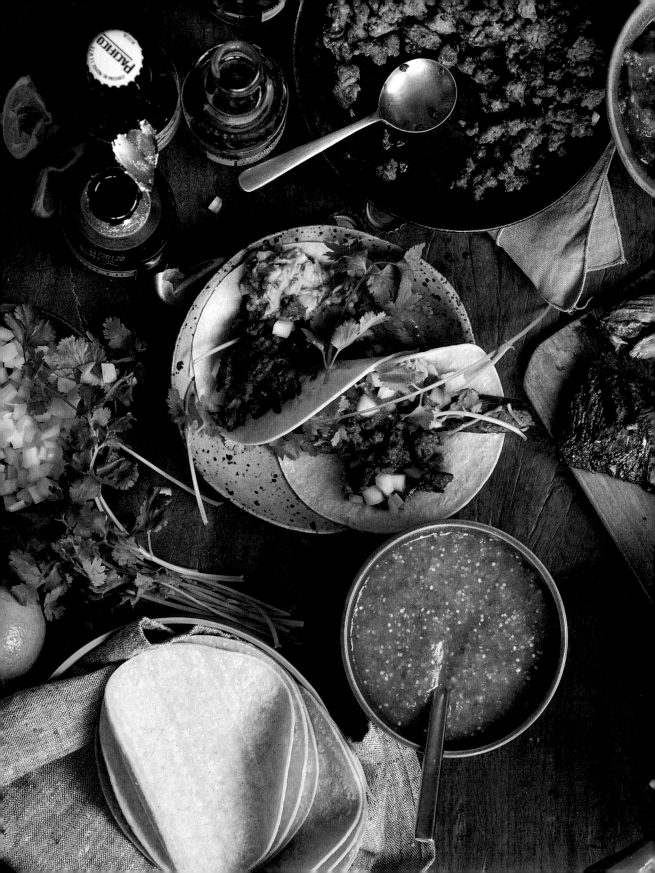

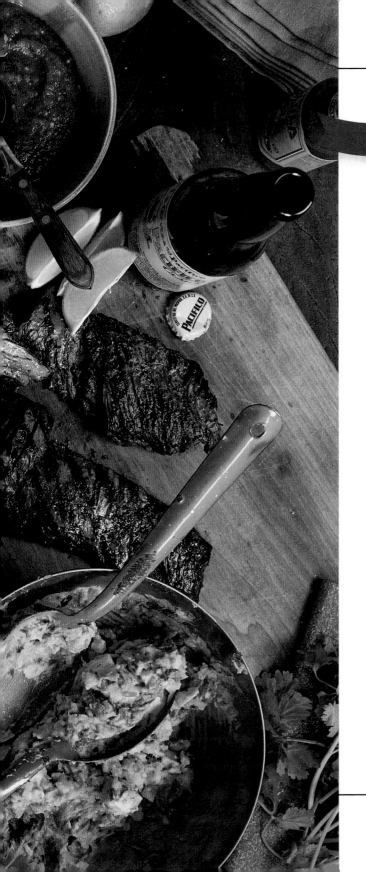

TACO NIGHT

You can do so much better than those "build-a-fiesta" boxes that amount to little more than a few stale hard shells and a packet of salty taco seasoning. In fact, you and your fellow eaters deserve more. We're talking fresh-tasting, cilantro-flecked guacamole. We're talking juicy seared skirt steak. We're talking lip-burning crumbled chorizo, green salsa with a bite, and slow-roasted pork carnitas. These are tacos that don't require gobs of sour cream or salty hot sauce packets to enjoy. Just top them with some diced onion and cilantro and you're set. Crack a cerveza. Chow down.

CARNE ASADA

Although it literally just means "grilled meat," *carne asada* is usually beef. Often the beef in question is *espaldilla* (boneless beef clod steak) or *diesmillo* (boneless beef chuck steak). At home, skirt steak or flank steak works just as well.

Juice of 2 lemons
6   tablespoons water
1   teaspoon garlic powder
1   scant teaspoon salt
1   pound skirt steak or flank steak
    Vegetable oil, for grilling

1. In a large resealable plastic bag, combine the lemon juice, water, garlic powder, and salt. Add the beef, massaging the marinade into the meat. Refrigerate for 1 to 3 hours.

2. Preheat a grill or grill pan to medium-high. (You should be able to hold your hand over it for no longer than 3 seconds.) Remove the meat from the marinade and pat it dry with paper towels. Lightly oil the hot grill and add the beef. Cook until the meat is nicely charred and the interior is just cooked through, about 3 minutes a side. Let rest a few minutes. Slice the beef into ½" strips and then hack it into nubs.

MAKES ENOUGH FOR 12 TACOS · PER SERVING/2 TACOS **150** CALORIES // **9 G** FAT // **439 MG** SODIUM // **2 G** CARBOHYDRATES // **0 G** DIETARY FIBER // **16 G** PROTEIN

CARNITAS

Usually made with pork, these "little meats" use a tough cut that turns amazingly tender as it simmers and then crisps up in its own fat. Carnitas are a fixture on the taco truck circuit. To play off the natural sweetness of the pork, pair it with salsa verde. This recipe comes courtesy of Chef Roberto Santibanez, chef/owner of Fonda restaurants in New York City.

2	pounds pork butt (shoulder), cut into 1½" chunks
1	tablespoon lard or vegetable oil
1½	cups water
½	orange, unpeeled and cut into 2 pieces
½	medium white onion, thinly sliced
4	cloves garlic, peeled
1	teaspoon dried oregano
1	teaspoon table salt or 2 teaspoons coarse salt
2	bay leaves

1. Combine all the ingredients in a 4- to 5-quart heavy pot; don't worry if the pork isn't completely covered. Bring everything to a boil, skimming as necessary. Then simmer rapidly over medium heat, stirring occasionally, until the pork is tender and the liquid has evaporated, about 1½ hours. Discard the orange and the bay leaves.

2. Continue to cook the pork in the fat left in the pan, stirring frequently, until it's golden brown, 10 to 15 minutes more.

MAKES ENOUGH FOR 16 TACOS · PER SERVING/2 TACOS 193 CALORIES // 10 G FAT // 379 MG SODIUM // 2 G CARBOHYDRATES // 1 G DIETARY FIBER // 22 G PROTEIN

MEXICAN CHORIZO

A sweetly aromatic pork sausage that's colored and perfumed with
paprika and other spices, chorizo is a nearly instant taco filling.
Find it alongside other fresh sausages in the meat case or at the butcher's.
(Don't confuse it with Spanish chorizo, which is a hard-cured, firm,
and ready-to-eat sausage.)

Remove the casings from 1 pound of Mexican chorizo links by cutting a slit along the length of each link
with a small, sharp knife. Then fry the chorizo over medium-high heat, breaking up the meat with a wooden
spoon, until it's cooked through and lightly browned, 5 to 8 minutes.

MAKES 12 SERVINGS · PER SERVING 172 CALORIES // **14 G** FAT // **467 MG** SODIUM // **1 G** CARBOHYDRATES //
0 G DIETARY FIBER // **9 G** PROTEIN

○ HEAT PERFECT TORTILLAS

The secret to taqueria-quality shells involves a dry pan. Heat a skillet (cast iron works best) on
medium-high. Add your tortilla and cook, turning every 10 seconds, until it's pliable. If you're in a
hurry, flick the flame of a gas stove to low and cook the tortilla directly on the burner.

THE ULTIMATE GUACAMOLE

The stuff from the tub is fine in a pinch, but only gringos depend on it. The best recipe for real guacamole is also the simplest, says Rick Bayless, executive chef of Frontera Grill in Chicago, Illinois.

1 PICK THE AVOCADO

Buy the pear-shaped, rough-skinned Hass variety. (Its texture is best.) If the fattest part yields slightly when you squeeze, it's good. If it's soft, has brittle skin, or the small button up top is gone, it's likely brown inside.

2 PREP THE ONION

Scoop the chopped onion into a strainer and run it under cold water for 30 seconds. This removes sulfurous compounds that can overpower the guacamole's taste.

3 MIX THE GUAC

Peel and dice 3 avocados. In a bowl, combine them with a small handful of chopped fresh cilantro, ½ cup chopped white onion, 1 minced jalapeño or serrano chile, a squeeze of lime juice, and salt to taste. Mix vigorously.

MAKES 6 SERVINGS · PER SERVING **168** CALORIES // **15 G** FAT // **58 MG** SODIUM // **10 G** CARBOHYDRATES // **7 G** DIETARY FIBER // **2 G** PROTEIN

○ PIT AND PEEL AN ADVOCADO

1 Insert a knife into the bottom of the avocado until the tip of the knife hits the pit.

2 Holding the knife stationary, rotate the avocado so that the blade cuts through the flesh all the way around, then twist the two halves to separate it.

3 Slide a spoon or a knife under the pit and pull it free. Cut the avocado into quarters, then pull off the skin.

TACO NIGHT

SALSA VERDE

Tomatillos, which look like green tomatoes with papery husks, give a sour edge to this salsa, while jalapeños add a dose of heat. Use this salsa to cut the richness of tacos made with carnitas or chorizo. It's also great with eggs and black beans.

10	fresh tomatillos, husks removed
1½	jalapeños, halved and seeded
½	cup fresh cilantro (leaves and stems)
½	small onion, chopped
2	cloves garlic
	Salt to taste

Add all the ingredients to a medium pot of boiling water. Reduce to a simmer and cook until softened, about 10 minutes. Let cool. Reserving 1 cup of the cooking liquid, drain the solids and transfer to a blender. Puree until mostly smooth. Season with salt and, if needed, thin with some of the reserved liquid.

MAKES ABOUT 2 CUPS (12 SERVINGS) ·
PER SERVING **12** CALORIES // **1 G** FAT // **14 MG** SODIUM //
2 G CARBOHYDRATES // **1 G** DIETARY FIBER // **1 G** PROTEIN

SALSA ROJA

The key to this salsa's intense, smoky flavor is char-roasted tomatoes and onions. It's especially good with carne asada. Make extra for tortilla chips—it'll keep in the fridge for a week.

6	medium tomatoes, halved
1	medium onion, quartered
2	cloves garlic
½	teaspoon dried oregano
½	teaspoon ground cumin
1	whole dried red chile or 1 teaspoon red-pepper flakes
	Salt to taste

1. Preheat the oven to 400°F. Line a baking sheet with foil. Place the tomatoes and onions on the pan and roast for 20 minutes. Then add the garlic and roast until the tomatoes collapse and begin to char, about 10 minutes more. (Watch the garlic; if it goes past blond, pull it.) Let cool.

2. In a dry skillet, toast the oregano, cumin, and chile over medium heat, stirring constantly, until fragrant, about 1 minute. Then puree all the ingredients in a blender until mostly smooth. Season with salt.

MAKES ABOUT 2 CUPS (12 SERVINGS) ·
PER SERVING **16** CALORIES // **1 G** FAT // **17 MG** SODIUM //
4 G CARBOHYDRATES // **1 G** DIETARY FIBER // **1 G** PROTEIN

BETTER-THAN-DELIVERY PIZZA

It's time to remove the pizza chain's number from your phone.

You can create healthier, tastier pie in less time than it takes for the pizza guy to ring your doorbell.

1

CREATE A PIZZA OVEN

To make crispy, evenly cooked, pizzeria-style pie, you'll need to jury-rig your oven. Crank the heat to its maximum setting (usually 500°F) and preheat two pizza stones or baking sheets, one on the top and one on the middle rack. The surfaces will help radiate heat around the pizza.

2

PREP THE CRUST

On a floured surface, stretch the dough to make a 12" to 14" crust. This works best if the dough is at room temperature. Don't worry if the pizza isn't perfectly round.

3

APPLY BASIC TOPPINGS

Transfer the crust to a floured pizza peel or pizza box lid. Spoon on your favorite jarred sauce or some crushed San Marzano canned tomatoes. Add slices of fresh mozzarella that you've patted dry.

4

PLACE IT IN THE OVEN

Slide the pie onto the middle rack's stone or sheet and bake until the crust is golden brown and the cheese is melted, 8 to 12 minutes.

5

ADD COLD TOPPINGS

Finish with easy, no-cook toppings (pick up to five): arugula, grated Parmigiano-Reggiano, grated Romano, goat cheese, Gorgonzola, red-pepper flakes, prosciutto, capicolla, fresh basil, fresh oregano. Then garnish with a drizzle of olive oil.

Meatballs

It's hard to imagine a food more primally pleasing than a well-made meatball. Few foods transcend geographic barriers as effectively and deliciously as the meatball does, and many of the world's food cultures have molded it to their culinary wills. The true genius of the meatball is its infinite versatility.

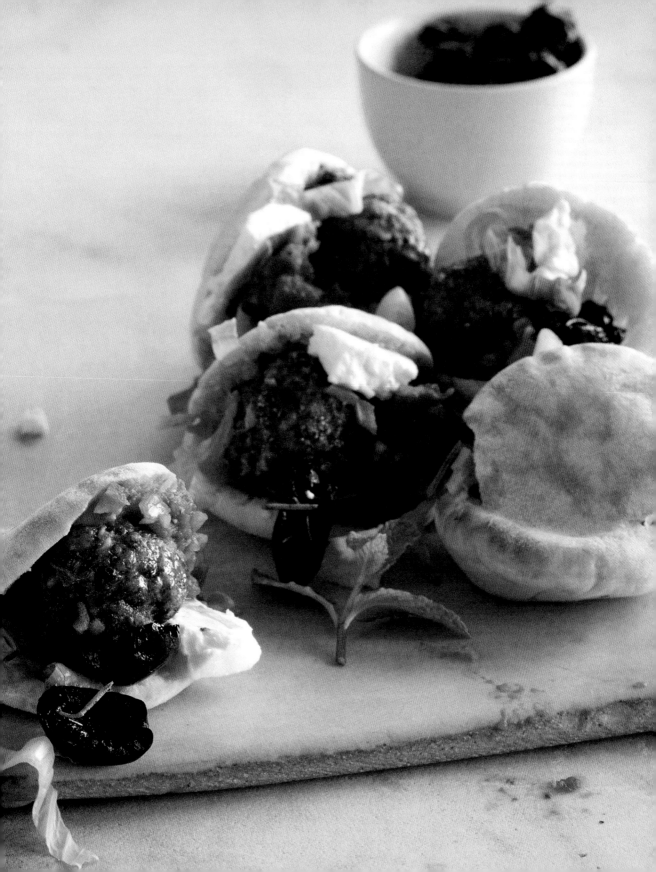

1 PICK YOUR PROTEIN

Meatballs can be made with nearly any ground protein: beef and pork, of course, but also duck, bison, lamb, or whatever else looks good in the meat case. Find a real butcher who's willing to run any cut of meat you want through the grinder. For 4 servings, start with 1½ pounds of meat or fish.

BEEF OR VEAL:	**CHICKEN OR TURKEY:**	**PORK OR SAUSAGE:**	**TUNA OR SALMON:**
Chuck has the ideal meat-to-fat ratio, but experiment with other cuts—brisket, sirloin, even short rib.	The milder flavors of chicken and turkey also work well in meatballs. For the best flavor, seek out dark meat instead of super-lean breast.	Use ground pork, or remove fresh sausage from its casing. Fresh chorizo works especially well for Mexican-style meatballs.	Remove the skin and bones, and pulse in a food processor until the flesh is reduced to small, pebble-size pieces.

2 ADD THE BINDER

Bread crumbs and eggs constitute the traditional one-two combo that holds meatballs together.

 2 large eggs $+$ ¾ cup unseasoned dry bread crumbs

3 SEASON THE MIXTURE

Seasonings form the flavor foundation and give your meatballs an identity.
Start with 1 teaspoon of salt and ½ teaspoon of ground black pepper, and then
experiment with one or more of the seasonings below.

| ½ cup minced onion | 1 tablespoon minced garlic | 1 tablespoon minced fresh ginger | 2 table-spoons minced jalapeño | 1 tablespoon grated citrus zest | ½ cup grated Parmesan or Romano cheese | ¼ cup chopped fresh herbs (or 1 teaspoon dried) |

4 COOK THE MEATBALLS

Form the meat mixture into 1"-diameter balls and arrange them on a baking tray.
Bake at 450°F until they're browned and caramelized, about 12 minutes.

5 PAIR WITH A SAUCE

All of these sauce recipes make 3 cups.

MUSHROOM GRAVY

Start by cooking your meatballs on the stove (don't bake them): In a large pan, brown the meatballs in batches over medium heat until cooked through, 10 to 12 minutes.

Transfer to a plate and add ½ pound sliced white mushrooms to the pan. Cook until browned, about 5 minutes. Stir in 2 tablespoons flour. Slowly whisk in 2 cups chicken broth. Then stir in ¼ cup heavy cream and simmer until the gravy has thickened, about 3 minutes.

MARINARA

In a medium saucepan, combine 2 tablespoons olive oil, ½ minced onion, 2 minced cloves garlic, and ¼ teaspoon red-pepper flakes. Cook over medium heat until the onion is soft, about 3 minutes.

Add a 28-ounce can whole tomatoes (with juice) and break up the tomatoes with a fork. Simmer until the sauce thickens, about 15 minutes. Season with salt and pepper.

MANGO CHUTNEY

In a medium saucepan, heat 1 tablespoon canola oil over medium heat. Add ½ diced red onion and 1 tablespoon each minced fresh ginger and garlic. Cook until soft, about 3 minutes. Add 1 diced mango, 1 diced red bell pepper, and 1 seeded and diced jalapeño pepper. Cook until the bell pepper is soft. Add ½ cup pineapple juice, 2 tablespoons red wine vinegar, and 1 tablespoon curry powder. Cook until thick, about 10 minutes.

SPICY LAMB MEATBALLS *with* TOMATO SAUCE, OLIVE, *and* FETA

These Greek-inspired meat orbs taste great on their own or tucked inside a pita with shredded lettuce for a kick-ass sandwich.

USE THIS PROTEIN

Lamb

USE THESE SEASONINGS

Onion

Garlic

1 teaspoon ground cumin

¼ teaspoon ground cinnamon

¼ teaspoon cayenne pepper

Mint

USE THIS SAUCE:

Marinara (see page 155)

MAKES 4 SERVINGS · PER SERVING **634** CALORIES // **39 G** FAT // **1,058 MG** SODIUM // **32 G** CARBOHYDRATES // **5 G** DIETARY FIBER // **40 G** PROTEIN

CLASSIC ITALIAN MEATBALLS *with* MARINARA SAUCE

Even if Grandma won't tell you her secret recipe, we will. All the perfect meatball takes is the right ingredients and a simple cooking treatment. No fuss. All good.

USE THIS PROTEIN

Equal parts beef, pork, and veal

USE THESE SEASONINGS

Parmesan

Parsley

USE THIS SAUCE:

Marinara (see page 155)

MAKES 4 SERVINGS · PER SERVING **557** CALORIES // **31 G** FAT // **1,399 MG** SODIUM // **26 G** CARBOHYDRATES // **3 G** DIETARY FIBER // **44 G** PROTEIN

ASIAN PORK MEATBALLS *with* MANGO CHUTNEY

Cook a big batch of these. You're going to want to eat them with a side of brown rice or soba noodles. Or for an awesome dinnertime sandwich, line them inside a whole wheat hoagie roll and top with sliced jalapeños and cilantro.

USE THIS PROTEIN
Pork

USE THESE SEASONINGS
Onion

Garlic

Ginger

Cilantro

USE THIS SAUCE:
Mango Chutney (see page 155)

MAKES 4 SERVINGS · PER SERVING **479** CALORIES // **15 G** FAT // **1,244 MG** SODIUM // **44 G** CARBOHYDRATES // **6 G** DIETARY FIBER // **40 G** PROTEIN

SWEDISH MEATBALLS *with* MUSHROOM GRAVY

Not only does Sweden export some of the world's loveliest supermodels, it has also given us the Swedish meatball, made with a mixture of beef and pork and coated in a rich gravy. Sweden, for these two things—models and meatballs—we forgive your long history of neutrality.

USE THIS PROTEIN
Equal parts beef and pork

USE THIS BINDER
Instead of dry bread crumbs, use 2 slices of white bread torn into small pieces and soaked in milk for 5 minutes. (Squeeze out the excess milk.)

USE THESE SEASONINGS
Onion

¼ teaspoon ground nutmeg

USE THIS SAUCE:
Mushroom Gravy (see page 155)

MAKES 4 SERVINGS · PER SERVING **391** CALORIES // **17 G** FAT // **1,223 MG** SODIUM // **15 G** CARBOHYDRATES // **1 G** DIETARY FIBER // **45 G** PROTEIN

MEAL-IN-A-BOWL BEEF SOUP

All sorts of vegetables work in this soup, so use whatever is fresh. Here are a few to start you thinking: tomatoes, pearl onions, potatoes, rutabagas or turnips, winter squash, or green beans. To make this soup a thick stew, just reduce the amount of stock by 2 cups or add more meat and vegetables.

2	tablespoons canola oil or corn oil
1	pound beef chuck or round, trimmed of external fat and cut into ½" cubes
1	onion, chopped
6	cups beef or other stock, or water
2	parsnips or carrots, peeled and diced
½	celeriac, peeled and diced, or 2 ribs celery, diced
1	cup diced butternut squash
2	sprigs of fresh thyme or rosemary
1	bay leaf
½	cup green peas (frozen are fine)
	Salt and ground black pepper
	Chopped fresh parsley leaves or chives

1. Heat the oil in a large, deep pot over medium-high heat. When it's hot, add the beef and cook until deeply browned on all sides, about 8 minutes. Pour off all but 2 tablespoons of the fat in the pan. Add the onion and cook until translucent, about 5 minutes.

2. Add the stock or water and bring to a near boil. Reduce the heat to a simmer, cover, and cook for 30 minutes. Add the parsnips or carrots, celeriac or celery, butternut squash, herb sprigs, and bay leaf, and stir. Cook until the meat and vegetables are tender, another 30 to 40 minutes.

3. Remove the herb sprigs and bay leaf and stir in the peas. Season with salt and pepper, taste, and adjust the seasoning. Serve garnished with parsley or chives.

MAKES 6 SERVINGS · PER SERVING **254** CALORIES // **12 G** FAT // **171 MG** SODIUM // **14 G** CARBOHYDRATES // **3 G** DIETARY FIBER // **22 G** PROTEIN

CHANGE IT UP

SPICY BEEF AND VEGETABLE SOUP Add 1 tablespoon of chopped garlic and 2 dried cascabel, guajillo, or pasilla chiles. Soak the chiles in just-boiled water for 10 minutes, drain them, and use a knife to scrape out the seeds and remove the stems. Then chop the chiles and add them along with the garlic to the cooked onions. For more kick, strain and add the chile soaking liquid (and reduce the amount of stock used).

BEEF AND MUSHROOM SOUP Add 4 cups chopped fresh mushrooms. Cook them along with the onion in step 1.

BETTER 'N MOM'S TOMATO SOUP

This soup delivers big health benefits, especially to men: lots of lycopene. Cooked tomatoes are one of the richest sources of lycopene, a carotenoid that is believed to lower the risk of prostate cancer, according to a study in the *Journal of the National Cancer Institute*. Put the canned tomato soup aside and learn how to make a pot of this delicious homemade concoction.

2	tablespoons extra-virgin olive oil
2	tablespoons tomato paste
1	large onion, sliced
1	carrot, diced
	Salt and ground black pepper
1	can (28 ounces) whole tomatoes
1	teaspoon fresh thyme leaves, ½ teaspoon dried thyme, or 1 tablespoon chopped fresh basil
3	cups chicken, beef, or vegetable stock, or water
1	teaspoon sugar (optional)
	Chopped fresh parsley or basil (optional)

1. Heat the oil in a large, deep pot over medium heat. Add the tomato paste and let it cook for a minute, then add the onion and carrot. Sprinkle with salt and pepper to taste and cook, stirring, until the onion begins to soften, about 5 minutes.

2. Add the tomatoes (with juice) and thyme or basil and cook, stirring occasionally, until the tomatoes break up, 10 to 15 minutes. Add the stock or water, stir, and cook until hot. Simmer for 5 minutes to meld the flavors. Taste and adjust the seasoning. If the soup tastes flat, stir in the sugar. If the mixture is too thick, add a little stock or water. Serve garnished with parsley or basil, if desired.

MAKES 4 SERVINGS · PER SERVING 172 CALORIES // 9 G FAT // 482 MG SODIUM // 18 G CARBOHYDRATES // 4 G DIETARY FIBER // 6 G PROTEIN

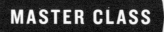

Essential Dips

Dips are notorious: salty, calorie-dense concoctions paired with carb-heavy dippers like potato chips, pretzels, and bagel chips. And most supermarket offerings have ingredient lists that read like a chemical spill. The homemade dips in this section taste better, are better for you, and require little work. And all come in under 200 calories per ⅓-cup serving.

SMOKY BLACK BEAN DIP

Most black bean dips are fairly healthful; the problem is that they often don't taste very good. This one employs ricotta for extra creaminess, prosciutto for a salty kick, chipotle for a hit of smokiness, and plenty of spices for layers of flavor.

1	can (15 ounces) black beans, rinsed and drained
1	cup low-fat ricotta
4	ounces prosciutto, chopped
	Juice of ½ lime
1	carrot, shredded
1	shallot or ¼ small red onion, chopped
1	tablespoon minced chipotle pepper in adobo sauce or 1 teaspoon smoked paprika
1	teaspoon ground cumin
1	teaspoon dried oregano
½	teaspoon salt

1. Place the beans in a food processor and pulse several times to break them up.

2. Add the ricotta, prosciutto, lime juice, carrot, shallot or onion, chipotle or paprika, cumin, oregano, and salt. Blend until smooth.

PER ⅓-CUP SERVING **74** CALORIES // **3 G** FAT // **521 MG** SODIUM // **8 G** CARBOHYDRATES // **2 G** DIETARY FIBER // **7 G** PROTEIN

CARAMELIZED ONION DIP

Who says you need a packet of soup mix to make an onion dip?
Actual caramelized onions lend savory depth to this dip, while protein-
filled Greek yogurt makes for smoother scooping.

1   tablespoon butter

2   large yellow onions, thinly
    sliced

1   tablespoon light brown
    sugar

1   teaspoon balsamic
    vinegar

3   cloves garlic, chopped

3   cups sliced mushrooms

¾   cup 2% Greek yogurt

1   tablespoon chopped fresh
    sage or rosemary

½   teaspoon salt

¼   teaspoon ground black
    pepper

1. Melt the butter in a large skillet over medium heat. Add the onions and cook until they soften, 4 to 5 minutes. Stir in the sugar and vinegar.

2. Reduce the heat to medium-low, cover, and cook for 25 minutes, stirring occasionally. Add the garlic and cook 5 minutes more. Transfer to a bowl.

3. Add the mushrooms to the same skillet. Increase the heat to medium and cook until tender, about 5 minutes.

4. Let the onions and mushrooms cool, and puree them in a food processor along with the yogurt, sage or rosemary, and salt.

PER ⅓-CUP SERVING **37** CALORIES // **1 G** FAT // **111 MG** SODIUM // **5 G** CARBOHYDRATES // **1 G** DIETARY FIBER // **2 G** PROTEIN

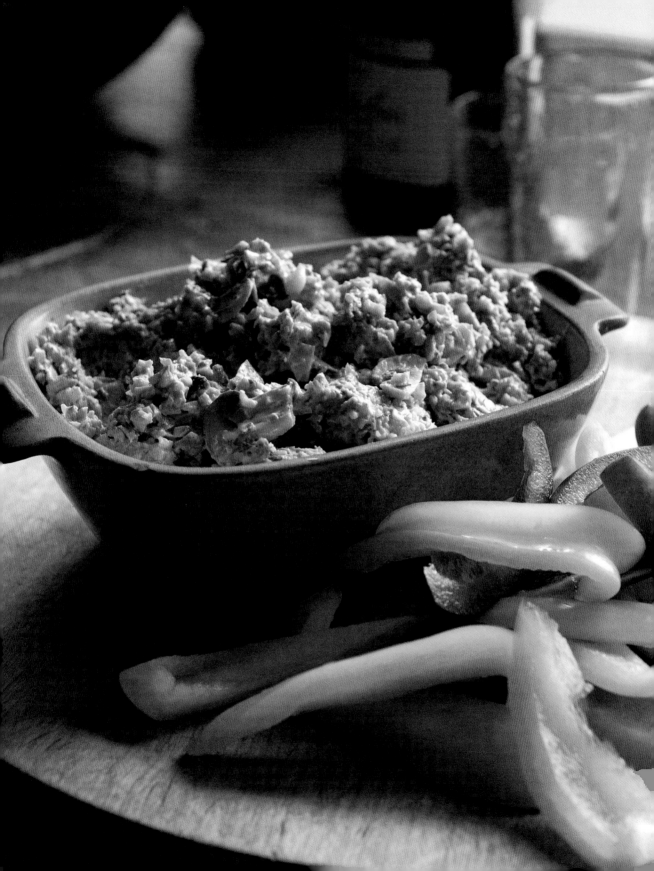

STOUT CHEESE DIP

It has beer. It has cheese. What more could a man possibly need?

2   cups shredded reduced-fat sharp cheddar cheese

1   shallot or ¼ small red onion, chopped

2   scallions, sliced

2   teaspoons grainy mustard

1   teaspoon prepared horseradish

1   tablespoon chopped fresh rosemary

¼   teaspoon salt

⅓   cup reduced-fat sour cream

¼   cup stout or dark beer (such as Guinness)

In a food processor, combine the cheddar, shallot or onion, scallions, mustard, horseradish, rosemary, and salt and pulse several times to combine. Add the sour cream and beer and blend until smooth.

PER ⅓-CUP SERVING **63** CALORIES // **3 G** FAT // **218 MG** SODIUM // **3 G** CARBOHYDRATES // **0 G** DIETARY FIBER // **6 G** PROTEIN

BETTER DIPPERS

Sure, standard tortilla chips do the job, but they won't score many points with a crowd. Instead, dip with a range of colorful, crunchy raw vegetables along with your choice of these alternative scoops.

SWEET POTATO FRIES

Lower in calories than most sweet potato chips. Try Alexia Sweet Potato Julienne Fries (alexiafoods.com).

PER 3-OUNCE SERVING:
140 CALORIES, 5 G FAT, 6 MG SODIUM, 8 G CARBOHYDRATES, 3 G DIETARY FIBER, 1 G PROTEIN

SMOKY LIME PITA CHIPS

Store-bought pita chips can be packed with excess oil. Best to bake your own instead: Slice 2 large whole-grain pitas into triangles and toss in a bowl with 1 tablespoon olive oil, the zest and juice of 1 lime, 1 teaspoon smoked paprika, and ½ teaspoon salt. Bake on a baking sheet at 350°F for 20 minutes, tossing once.

PER 1-PITA SERVING:
240 CALORIES, 9 G FAT, 931 MG SODIUM, 38 G CARBOHYDRATES, 5 G DIETARY FIBER, 7 G PROTEIN

JERKY

Packed with hunger-quelling protein. Try venison, elk, or even ostrich. You can even make your own—see page 76.

PER 1-OUNCE SERVING:
65 CALORIES, 8 G FAT, 474 MG SODIUM, 2 G CARBOHYDRATES, 12 G PROTEIN

JOHNNIE'S ITALIAN BEEF

Johnnie's Italian beef, a Chicago-area sandwich shop, serves its namesake on a thick Italian roll and piles it with sliced beef, a sluice of gravy, and giardiniera, a medley of pickled Italian vegetables. Taste one, become a convert. And then, because the recipe makes seven more servings, share.

6   **cloves garlic, thinly sliced**
3   **pounds boneless chuck roast**
1   **cup water**
2   **bay leaves**
1   **tablespoon red-pepper flakes**
1   **tablespoon dried oregano**
2   **teaspoons salt**
1   **tablespoon coarsely ground black pepper**
8   **small Italian rolls, split and toasted**

1. Preheat the oven to 250°F. Use a small knife to insert the garlic slivers all over the roast.

2. Pour the water into a deep baking pan not much larger than the roast. Add the roast and all the seasonings. Cover tightly and bake for 2 hours, basting three or four times.

3. Remove the beef from the pan and let it rest for about 15 minutes. With an extremely sharp knife, slice it into razor-thin pieces.

4. Skim the excess fat from the juices in the pan. They should be highly seasoned, with a peppery bite. Adjust the seasoning and place the sliced beef in the juices. Let the beef wallow 15 to 20 minutes. Serve on the Italian rolls with either giardiniera or roasted sweet peppers.

MAKES 8 SERVINGS · PER SERVING (WITH ROLL) 445 CALORIES // 11 G FAT // 1,049 MG SODIUM // 40 G CARBOHYDRATES // 4 G DIETARY FIBER // 45 G PROTEIN

CHICKEN-AND-SAUSAGE STEW
with GREENS *and* WHITE BEANS

Maybe the word "stew" conjures up memories of Mom's dump-and-cook casseroles. Allow Chef Brandon Boudet, of Dominick's in Los Angeles, California, to change your mind. Hearty kale and cannellini beans stand up to the dark-meat chicken and spicy sausage, coming together in a stick-to-your-ribs recipe that won't bust your gut.

4	boneless, skinless chicken thighs, halved
	Coarse salt
	Red-pepper flakes
¼	cup extra-virgin olive oil
¾	pound andouille sausage, sliced
1	yellow onion, chopped
2	carrots, sliced into ¼" rounds
4	cloves garlic, smashed
1	tablespoon fennel seeds
8	cups low-sodium chicken broth
1	can (15 ounces) cannellini beans, rinsed and drained
1	bunch kale, trimmed and chopped
	Juice of 1 lemon

1. Season the chicken with salt and pepper flakes to taste.

2. Preheat an 8-quart pot over medium-high heat, then add 2 tablespoons of the olive oil. Add the thighs and cook without turning until they're seared on one side, about 3 minutes. Turn them and add the sausage. Cook about 5 minutes more. Stir the sausage occasionally until it's browned.

3. Add the onion, carrots, garlic, and fennel seeds and cook until the onion is translucent, about 8 minutes. Add the broth and bring it to a boil. Add the beans, reduce the heat to low, cover, and simmer until the chicken is cooked through, about 40 minutes.

4. Add the kale and simmer uncovered, adding more broth if the stew looks too thick, until the ingredients are tender, about 30 minutes more. Stir in the remaining 2 tablespoons oil and the lemon juice, and season with more pepper flakes and salt.

MAKES 6 SERVINGS · PER SERVING 419 CALORIES // 24 G FAT // 828 MG SODIUM // 25 G CARBOHYDRATES // 5 G DIETARY FIBER // 31 G PROTEIN

Chicken

When in doubt, roast a chicken, says Mark Bittman, author of *How to Cook Everything: The Basics*. A whole bird, seasoned simply with just salt and pepper (and maybe some lemon halves), undergoes an alchemy in the oven, emerging much more delicious than the sum of its parts. But don't stop there. The mild flavor of chicken is a blank slate that will take on any seasoning. And you can use that roast chicken as a jumping-off point to a range of easy meals.

1 COOK THE BIRD

Start with a whole chicken, giblets removed. Position a rack in the lower third of the oven. Put a large ovenproof skillet on the rack and preheat to 400°F.

GIVE IT A RUB

While the oven preheats, trim the excess fat from the bird. Pat dry with paper towels. Rub the bird with 3 tablespoons of olive oil and sprinkle it with salt and black pepper. Place three lemon halves in the cavity. (See "Customize It" on page 170.)

When the pan is scorching hot, 10 to 15 minutes later, carefully add the chicken, breast-side up. Roast until the chicken is cooked through (it should register 155° to 165°F on a meat thermometer), 40 to 60 minutes, depending on its size.

USE THE JUICE

Carefully remove the pan from the oven. Tip the pan to let any juices from the bird's cavity flow into the pan, then transfer the chicken to a cutting board.

Let the pan juices sit until the fat rises to the top, about 5 minutes, then use a spoon to skim off some of the excess fat. Cut the bird and serve it with the warm pan juices.

2 ACHIEVE PERFECT DONENESS

While undercooked chicken is always a concern, it's also important not to overcook the bird. A few tips will help you target the temperature.

HIT THE MARK

The internal temperature of the meat varies depending on where you test it. Always test doneness in the thickest part of the thigh, since that part of the chicken takes the longest to cook.

IMPROVISE IF NECESSARY

An instant-read meat thermometer is the most reliable way to test doneness, but if you don't have one, try the "cut and run" method: Pierce a chicken thigh all the way to the bone with a paring knife. If clear juices run out, the chicken's done. If the juices are reddish or pink, the bird's not ready yet.

REMEMBER THE RISE

The USDA recommends that you cook chicken to at least 160°F to avoid any risk of foodborne illness. But a roast chicken will continue to cook (from residual heat) even after it comes out of the oven, so it's fine to remove it when the internal temperature reads 155°F.

MAKES 4 SERVINGS · PER SERVING **594** CALORIES // **23 G** FAT // **379 MG** SODIUM // **0 G** CARBOHYDRATES // **0 G** DIETARY FIBER // **92 G** PROTEIN

3 MAKE A MEAL

BBQ SANDWICH

Caramelize sliced onions in some olive oil, then toss in shredded chicken and good barbecue sauce and cook, stirring, until heated through. Serve on a roll or in a wrap with shredded lettuce, cabbage, or coleslaw if you've got some.

TORTILLA SOUP

Pull the chicken meat from the bones. Put the carcass in a large pot with a halved onion and a few bay leaves, and cover with water. Simmer until flavorful, about 30 minutes; season with salt and pepper. Strain the broth, add the chicken pieces, and heat through. Ladle into bowls and top with crumbled feta; tortilla chips; and chopped tomato, radishes, and/or avocado.

CURRIED CHICKEN SALAD

Mix shredded chicken with a combo of mayo, plain yogurt, chopped cilantro, and chopped red onion, seasoned with a dash of curry powder, salt, and pepper. Fold in diced apples and whole cashews, if you like. Serve on crackers or bread with any kind of chutney.

CHICKEN QUESADILLA

Stir together some shredded chicken, grated cheese, and chopped red onion; add chili powder to taste. Spread the mixture between 2 flour or corn tortillas. Brush with olive oil and grill, broil, or pan-fry, turning once. Cut into wedges and serve with lime wedges.

○ CUSTOMIZE IT

SAVORY HERB
Put a few sprigs of fresh herbs—like rosemary, thyme, parsley, or sage—in the chicken's cavity. Or sprinkle the skin with up to 1 teaspoon dried or minced fresh herbs, like thyme or oregano.

MISO-GARLIC
Gently coat the skin of the chicken with a mixture of white miso and minced garlic. If you're ambitious, carefully separate the skin from the meat with your fingers and rub the seasoning in between.

SOY-SESAME
Use vegetable oil instead of olive oil to coat the chicken, and stir a dash of soy sauce and sesame oil into the pan juices.

MAKE CHICKEN CHEAPER

Another way to make chicken more versatile—and save money, too—is to learn to break down a bird into parts for individual meals. A whole chicken is cheaper than a precut one, so dissecting it yourself can net you more nutrients per dollar.

1
REMOVE THE WINGS

Keep the blade flat against the chicken, and then slide it into the bird's "armpit" until you hit bone. Find the joint and cut through the cartilage.

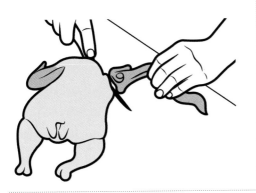

2
CUT OFF THE LEGS

Slice into the hip and bend the leg up to pop the joint. Cut through the cartilage and pull off the leg along with the backbone meat. Slice off the thighs above the drumstick.

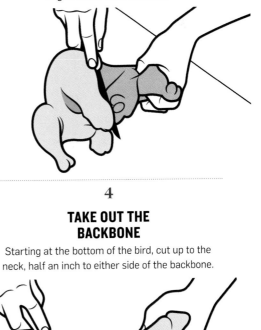

3
SEPARATE THE BREAST

Make a shallow cut down the center of the inner chest membrane. Push the sternum up from underneath with your fingers and pull it out completely. Cut the breast in half.

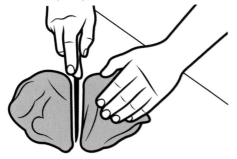

4
TAKE OUT THE BACKBONE

Starting at the bottom of the bird, cut up to the neck, half an inch to either side of the backbone.

MAKE CHICKEN SOUP FROM SCRATCH

There's a reason why your mom's chicken soup was so much more soul-satisfying than the stuff from a can.

1 BUY THE RIGHT BIRD

A 3- to 4-pound roaster (an older bird) will give your soup a strong chicken flavor and leave you with plenty of extra meat for leftovers.

2 SALT THE MEAT

For tastier soup, rub the chicken inside and out with 1 tablespoon of kosher salt, and refrigerate for 15 minutes. Then rinse the bird with cold water and pat dry.

3 PREP THE VEGETABLES

Aromatic vegetables add a foundation of flavor.

BEST MIX:

3 carrots + 5 ribs celery + 1 onion + 3 cloves garlic
(CHOPPED)　　　(CHOPPED)　　　(CHOPPED)　　　(WHOLE, PEELED)

4 GATHER YOUR SEASONINGS

For a classic chicken soup, stick to subtle herbs and spices.

BEST MIX:

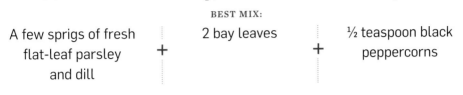

A few sprigs of fresh flat-leaf parsley and dill

+

2 bay leaves

+

½ teaspoon black peppercorns

5 COOK THE SOUP

A. Place the bird in a large pot and add enough water to cover it by 3 inches. Bring to a boil and skim off any foam.

B. Add the vegetables and seasonings. Simmer, uncovered, until the chicken is cooked, about 45 minutes.

C. Transfer the chicken to a large bowl. When it's cool enough to handle, strip the meat from the bones, discarding the skin.

D. Return the bones to the pot and simmer for another hour. Strain the broth (discard the solids) and season with salt and pepper.

6 CHOOSE YOUR ADD-INS

Cooked egg noodles | brown or wild rice | canned white beans | fresh baby spinach | chopped dill or parsley

7 MAKE IT BETTER

For a clearer, less greasy broth, refrigerate it overnight.
The next day, skim off the solidified fat and reheat.

PAIR BEER *to* FOOD

"Good food can make good beer taste better, and vice versa," says Aviram Turgeman, a beer sommelier at Café D'Alsace in Manhattan.

1

PIZZA OR MACKEREL
+
PILSNER, LAGER

WHY IT WORKS Structure
A dry, crisp beer with balanced hops can balance rich and gamey flavors. Plus, the hops can scrub your taste buds between bites, enhancing the flavor of both beer and food.

TURGEMAN'S PICK Jever Pilsener
Also try . . . Stella Artois, Kronenbourg 1664

2

BURGER, CHICKEN, OR LAMB
+
AMBER ALE

WHY IT WORKS Intensity
"Strong flavors overwhelm light beers," says Turgeman. That's why you need a complex, heavier brew.

TURGEMAN'S PICK Fischer Amber
Also try . . . Sierra Nevada Pale Ale, Samuel Smith's Nut Brown Ale

3

BEEF, SAUSAGE, OR PORK
+
FARMHOUSE ALE

WHY IT WORKS Region
European beers taste great with meat cooked in European styles. Carry the lesson to other cuisines, to complement undertones in each: Asian beer with sushi, a Mexican cerveza with tacos, and so on.

TURGEMAN'S PICK Saison Dupont
Also try . . . La Choulette Blonde, Castelain Blond

4

GREEN SALAD OR EGG
+
BELGIAN WHITE

WHY IT WORKS Weight/body
Citrus-packed, lighter wheat beers make food taste fresher and cut through the richness of salad dressing or hollandaise sauce.

TURGEMAN'S PICK Gruut Belgian Wit Beer
Also try . . . Hoegaarden, Blue Moon

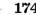

5

CHEESE OR SALMON
+
TRAPPIST, ABBEY

WHY IT WORKS Body/strength

The mild sweetness and yeastiness of Trappist beers play off the richness of smoked or grilled food or pungent cheese.

TURGEMAN'S PICK Chimay Red

Also try . . . Leffe Blonde, Goose Island Matilda

6

CHOCOLATE OR FRUIT
+
STOUT, PORTER, FLAVORED LAMBICS

WHY IT WORKS There are no rules

"Experiment with sweet beers," Turgeman says. "You can make great combinations." To cap off a dinner date, pair chocolate with cherry lambic.

TURGEMAN'S PICK Lindemans Kriek Lambic

Also try . . . Smuttynose Robust Porter, Young's Double Chocolate Stout

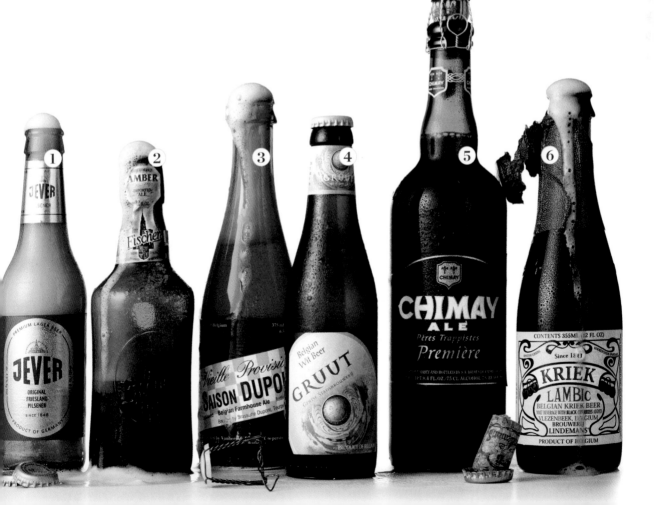

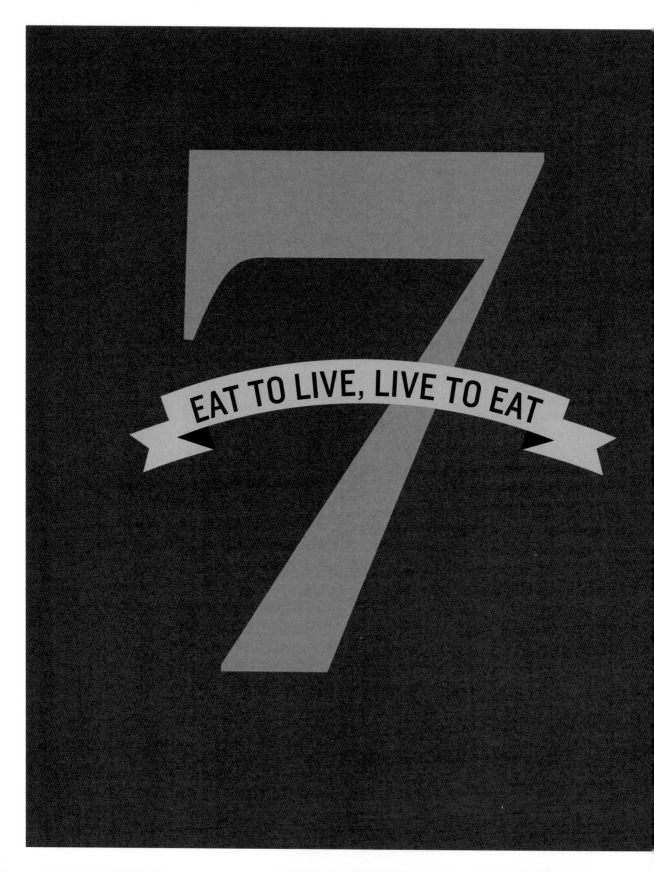

EATING OUTSIDE

From grilling to barbecuing to camp cookery, here's how to make yourself the lord of the fires.

GUY
MH
GOURMET

p. 178   c. 07

READY, SET, GRILL

When man cooked his first steak, it must have been a beautiful thing. One can understand the mechanical importance of The Wheel, or the powerful nature of The Spear, but when man touched meat to flame, what could have been more visceral, more earth-stopping than The Steak? Honor your fire-starting forebearers with the recipes that follow, using these integral rules for better grilling. Let there be fire.

RULE Nᴼ·

1

LIGHT THE GRILL

IF YOU HAVE a gas grill, crank the heat and skip to Rule No. 2. If you have a charcoal grill, skip the lighter fluid—it gives your food a funky smell and taste. Instead, use a chimney starter, available at any hardware or kitchen store for about $15. Stuff a sheet or two of newspaper into the bottom of the chimney, set the chimney on the grill grates, and fill it with hardwood charcoal (briquettes are cheaper and easier to find, but they have chemical binders that affect your food's taste). Light the newspaper and watch for smoke to emerge from the top of the chimney. In about 15 minutes, your coals will be lightly covered with ash—a sign that they're ready to go. Hold the chimney with a heatproof glove or with a heavy dish towel, and shake out the coals into your grill.

RULE № 2 | SCRUB THE GRATES

CLOSE THE GRILL lid and leave it for 3 to 5 minutes. The high temperature will char any food residue so it's easier to scrape off. Then remove the charred residue from the grates with a semiflexible stainless steel brush.

RULE № 3 | CREATE A COOKING ZONE

DIRECT HEAT If you're cooking thinner cuts of meat like chicken breasts, pork chops, steaks, and burgers, dump your hot coals in the center of the grill (or light all the burners on your gas grill) and allow the grates to heat. Arrange the meat directly above the coals on the grate. Cook with the lid open.

INDIRECT HEAT If you're cooking whole chickens, whole turkeys, rib roasts, and other larger pieces of meat that would burn if you used direct grilling, or if you want to infuse big, tough cuts with plenty of smoky flavor and tenderness, go low and slow. If you're using a kettle grill, you'll need to create an indirect heat zone in the center of your grill using a technique called "banking." Using a grill hoe or a pair of long metal tongs, push the coals to the edges of your grill, leaving an open space in the center. If you're using a bullet smoker, just add the hot coals to the bottom of the cooker. To add smoke, wrap your presoaked wood chunks or chips in foil, poke some large holes in the package, and toss directly onto the hot coals. If you're using a gas grill, turn the burners on one side of the grill to low; use the opposite side of the grill for cooking.

RULE № 4 | REGULATE THE HEAT

TO TEST YOUR grill heat, place your hand 3 inches above the grates and count "one Mississippi . . ." until you have to pull away. Less than 3 seconds is high heat; 5 to 6 is medium; 10 to 12 is low. To lower the heat, vent the grill or open the lid for a minute or two. To raise the heat, add 4 to 6 more lit coals, one at a time. (Keep a supply on hand in the chimney starter.) And remember, the sweet spot for barbecue is between 225° and 250°F. A low, even heat will help break down the collagen in the muscles and create tender meat.

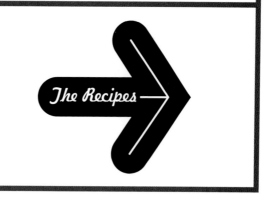

The Recipes →

GEAR

5 GRILLING TOOLS EVERY MAN SHOULD OWN

Meat? Check. Grill? Fired up. Sear spear?

To make the most tender, mouthwatering slab possible, you'll need the right tools. Upgrade your outdoor cooking routine with this streamlined guide.

 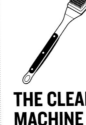 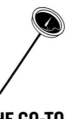 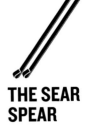

THE SAUCE SLINGER

Skip silicone basting brushes, which are easy to clean but don't hold enough sauce. We like ones with natural bristles, or use a mop brush with thick string, which can slather sauce quickly.

THE CLEAN MACHINE

The cleaner your grate is, the better contact your meat will have for searing and well-defined grill marks. Plus, you won't taste last summer's cheeseburgers.

THE FAST FLIPPER

As you're grilling, you should move the meat only three times: to put it on the heat, to flip it, and to remove it. Prodding and pushing dries it out. So instead of chasing your dinner around the grate with a spatula, use long-reach grill tongs.

THE GO-TO GAUGE

No knives at the grill! Cutting meat to test doneness spills juices, leaving the meat tough and dry. Buy a digital instant read meat thermometer and use our temperature guide (see page 18).

THE SEAR SPEAR

Thin skewers have a tendency to crawl around grill grates, spinning to their heavy sides. Wide, swordlike skewers stabilize kebabs by adding heft, meaning you only have to turn them once while grilling. Their heavier weight also makes them perfect for lancing large hunks of meat and chunks of vegetables.

BALSAMIC LAMB CHOPS

Think of them as meat popsicles. Grill them
and then eat them straight off the bone.

---

2   tablespoons olive oil

2   cloves garlic, minced

1   tablespoon finely chopped fresh rosemary

1   pound lamb rib chops

½   cup balsamic vinegar

    Salt and black pepper, to taste

1. In a small bowl, whisk together the oil, garlic, and three-fourths of the chopped rosemary. Place the lamb chops in a resealable plastic bag and pour the marinade over them. Seal the bag and refrigerate for up to 4 hours.

2. Combine the remaining rosemary and the balsamic vinegar in a small saucepan set over medium heat. Cook until the vinegar reduces by about three-fourths. (It should easily coat the back of a spoon.) Set aside.

3. Preheat a grill to high. When it's very hot, season the lamb chops all over with salt and pepper and grill for 2 to 3 minutes per side, until the meat is firm but still yielding. Serve with the balsamic syrup drizzled over the chops.

MAKES 4 SERVINGS · PER SERVING **280** CALORIES // **21 G** FAT // **435 MG** SODIUM // **0 G** CARBOHYDRATES // **0 G** DIETARY FIBER // **23 G** PROTEIN

✚ KITCHEN EMT ✚
ZING THAT STING

Stung by a yellow jacket while grilling steaks? Work up a paste of meat tenderizer with a few drops of water and apply it to the sting. (Flick the stinger out of your skin first with a fingernail.) The enzymes in the tenderizer break down the offending venom that turns your skin red.

CEDAR-PLANK SALMON

Dilemma: You love the taste of smoked foods but you don't have enough time to slow-cook dinner in your barbecue rig. Solution: Pick up a cedar plank from the grilling section of your supermarket and use its subtle smoky flavor to infuse the fish it'll support throughout the grilling process.

1	large, untreated cedar plank
1	large English (hothouse) cucumber, seeded and sliced
2	tablespoons rice vinegar
1	teaspoon red-pepper flakes
2	teaspoons sesame seeds, plus more for garnish
2	tablespoons chopped fresh mint or cilantro
	Salt and ground black pepper
	Olive oil
2	salmon fillets (6 ounces each)

1. Soak the cedar plank in water for at least 2 hours.

2. In a bowl, combine the cucumber, vinegar, pepper flakes, sesame seeds, and mint or cilantro. Season with salt and black pepper to taste.

3. Rub the grates with an oil-soaked paper towel. Fire up the grill to high. Lay the cedar plank on the grill. Season the salmon with salt and pepper. When the plank begins to smoke, lay the fillets on it, skin side down. Close the top, and grill until the salmon flakes with light pressure from your finger, 10 to 12 minutes.

4. Serve the salmon topped with the cucumbers, and garnish with a sprinkling of sesame seeds.

MAKES 2 SERVINGS · PER SERVING 300 CALORIES // 12 G FAT // 200 MG SODIUM // 8 G CARBOHYDRATES // 2 G DIETARY FIBER // 36 G PROTEIN

GRILL A WHOLE FISH

Feeding the family or a group of friends? Don't rule out fish because it's too tricky. Simplify your approach by flopping the entire fish on the grill.

THE FISH

To feed 6, you'll need 4 pounds of whole fish (two 2-pounders or four 1-pounders)—red snapper, striped bass, porgie, or mackerel—cleaned and scaled. Leave the head, fins, and tail on for visual impact.

THE FLAVORING

Season the fish inside and out with salt, and brush the skin with extra-virgin olive oil (garlic-infused, if possible). Then stuff (don't overstuff) the cavity with your choice of aromatics—thinly sliced garlic or onion, sprigs of thyme or rosemary, slices of lemon or orange.

THE TECHNIQUE

Heat your grill to medium-high (425° to 450°F). Once it's hot, lightly oil the grate and lay the fish directly on it. Cook without moving until a crust forms and the fish lifts easily, about 15 minutes. Turn the fish using a wide spatula, and cook until the flesh flakes when lightly prodded with a fork, about 10 minutes more.

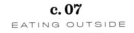

GRILLED TUNA
with SAUCE VIERGE

Just because they're called tuna steaks doesn't mean you should treat them like a porterhouse. Tuna cooks faster than beef or pork and deserves a lighter treatment on the finish. Go with sauce vierge, says Eric Ripert, executive chef of Le Bernardin in New York City. (That's a fancy way to say "a simple sauce with olive oil and tomatoes as its base.") Sauce vierge also keeps well in the fridge for at least 3 days, and with a little acid can be used as a great vinaigrette.

½   cup extra-virgin olive oil

    Grated zest of 1 lemon

2   tablespoons lemon juice

½   pint cherry tomatoes, quartered

1   small shallot, minced

½   clove garlic, minced

3   tablespoons chopped parsley

    Fine sea salt and ground black pepper

4   tuna steaks, about 1" thick

4   tablespoons herbes de Provence

¼   cup olive oil

1. Fire up the grill to high.

2. In a medium bowl, combine the extra-virgin olive oil, lemon zest, lemon juice, tomatoes, shallot, garlic, and parsley. Season with salt and pepper to taste. Set aside.

3. When the grill is ready, season the tuna generously with the herbes de Provence, salt, and pepper.

4. Drizzle the olive oil over the fish and place it on the grill. Sear for 2 to 3 minutes on each side for medium-rare (an internal temp of 110°F), and serve immediately with the sauce.

MAKES 4 SERVINGS · PER SERVING **703** CALORIES // **57 G** FAT // **815 MG** SODIUM // **7 G** CARBOHYDRATES // **1 G** DIETARY FIBER // **40 G** PROTEIN

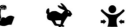

GRILLED FISH TACOS
with CHIPOTLE CREMA

Fried fish tacos on menus at sit-down chains usually come clobbered with fried batter to make up for tasteless fish. Avoid the calorie overload by using better-quality fish and fresh toppings like cabbage and avocado.

½	cup Mexican crema or sour cream
3	limes—1 juiced, 2 cut into wedges
1	tablespoon finely chopped canned chipotle pepper in adobo sauce
	Chopped fresh cilantro
	Vegetable oil, for the grill
1	pound mahi-mahi, halibut, or fresh tuna
1½	teaspoons chile powder (preferably ancho)
	Salt and ground black pepper
8	corn tortillas
1	cup finely shredded cabbage
1	avocado, thinly sliced
	Hot sauce

1. Fire up the grill to medium-high.

2. In a small bowl, mix together the crema with the lime juice, chipotle, and a handful of chopped fresh cilantro. Set aside.

3. Drizzle a light coating of oil over the fish and rub on the chile powder and a pinch each of salt and black pepper. Place the fish on the grill and cook, undisturbed, for 4 minutes. Carefully flip it with a spatula and cook for another 4 minutes. Remove. Before turning off the grill, warm the tortillas directly on the surface for 1 to 2 minutes.

4. Divide the fish evenly among the warm tortillas, add a bit of cabbage, spoon on the crema mixture, and top with avocado slices and fresh cilantro. Serve each taco with a wedge of lime and some hot sauce.

MAKES 8 TACOS · PER SERVING (2 TACOS) **363** CALORIES // **16 G** FAT // **208 MG** SODIUM // **33 G** CARBOHYDRATES // **8 G** DIETARY FIBER // **25 G** PROTEIN

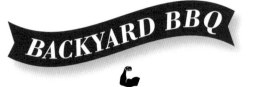

BACKYARD BABY BACKS

Barbecue barons John Stage of Dinosaur BBQ in Syracuse, New York,
and Kenny Callaghan of Blue Smoke in Manhattan deliver
the ultimate ribs recipe with their signature sauce made exclusively
for *Men's Health*. The work is worth it.

3	cups wood chips (apple or cherry)
2	slabs (2 pounds each) baby-back or loin-back ribs
	Rib Rub (page 188)
¼	cup pineapple juice
	Real BBQ Sauce (page 188)

1. Soak the wood chips for 20 minutes and drain. Fire up the grill for indirect heat and add the wood. Fill a large aluminum foil pan with ⅛" water. Remove the grill grate, place the pan next to the coals (or the heat source for gas grills), and replace the grate.

2. Coat the ribs on both sides with ¼ cup of the rib rub. Place the ribs opposite the fire, over the water pan. Cover and cook at 250°F for 2 hours.

3. Remove the ribs and place each rack on a large sheet of foil. Add 2 tablespoons of pineapple juice to each rack, wrap them tightly, and return them to the grill. Continue to cook the ribs until the meat begins to loosen from the bone, 45 to 60 minutes.

4. Meanwhile, make the Real BBQ Sauce.

5. Remove the ribs from the foil and return them to the grill, sprinkling them lightly with more rub. Cook the ribs for 20 more minutes, and then brush the BBQ sauce on both sides. Keep cooking the meat until it tears easily between the bones and the rack bends when you hold it in the middle with tongs, another 25 to 40 minutes.

MAKES 8 SERVINGS · PER SERVING **917** CALORIES // **72 G** FAT // **518 MG** SODIUM // **14 G** CARBOHYDRATES // **0 G** DIETARY FIBER // **49 G** PROTEIN

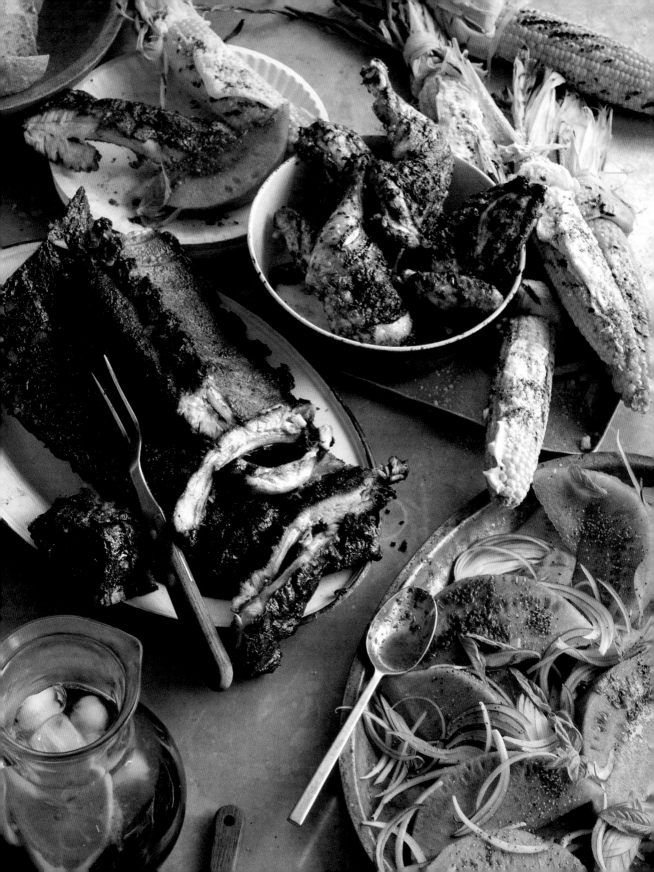

BACKYARD BBQ

RIB RUB

- ¼ cup paprika
- ¼ cup kosher salt
- ¼ cup dark brown sugar
- 2½ tablespoons granulated garlic
- 2 tablespoons granulated onion
- 2 tablespoons chili powder
- 1 tablespoon coarsely ground black pepper
- 2 teaspoons ground cumin
- ½ teaspoon cayenne pepper

In a medium bowl, combine all the ingredients.

MAKES ABOUT 1 CUP

REAL BBQ SAUCE

This stuff is so much better than the bottled sauce, you'll be reaching for a straw. This recipe makes a lot; share a jar with a friend or refrigerate what you don't use. It'll keep in the fridge up to a month.

- 2 tablespoons vegetable oil
- ½ cup minced onion
- ¼ cup minced green bell pepper
- ½ jalapeño pepper, seeded and minced
- 1 tablespoon minced garlic
- Pinch of kosher salt
- 1 can (15 ounces) tomato sauce
- 1 cup ketchup
- ½ cup honey
- ½ cup water
- 6 tablespoons dark brown sugar
- 6 tablespoons Worcestershire sauce
- ¼ cup cider vinegar
- 2 tablespoons lemon juice
- 2 tablespoons molasses
- 2 tablespoons sambal chili sauce
- 2 tablespoons cayenne-pepper sauce, such as Frank's RedHot
- 2 tablespoons spicy brown mustard
- 1½ teaspoons chili powder
- 1 teaspoon coarsely ground black pepper
- ¼ teaspoon ground allspice
- 1½ teaspoons liquid smoke (optional)

Heat the oil in a large saucepan over medium-high heat. Add the onion, bell pepper, jalapeño, and garlic, cooking them until soft, about 10 minutes. Add the remaining ingredients and bring the mixture to a boil, stirring occasionally. Pour the sauce into a container.

MAKES ABOUT 5 CUPS

REAL JERK CHICKEN

Think you know barbecue chicken? This spicy, smoky chicken is the next step in your pitmaster evolution. Jerk relies on low, indirect heat to slow-cook the meat to tenderness and allow the spices to infuse every bite. Try this recipe, by Darren Lee, chef of the Strawberry Hill Hotel and Spa in Jamaica, and you'll never turn back. Bonus: You'll have plenty of jerk paste left over for your next batch.

5	scallions, coarsely chopped
2	Scotch bonnet chiles, roughly chopped
2	cloves garlic, roughly chopped
¼	cup distilled white vinegar
2	tablespoons vegetable oil
5½	teaspoons kosher salt
2	teaspoons ground allspice
2	teaspoons ground cinnamon
2	teaspoons finely chopped fresh thyme
1½	teaspoons finely chopped fresh ginger
1	teaspoon light brown sugar
1	teaspoon ground black pepper
1	teaspoon ground nutmeg
3½-	to 4-pound chicken, cut into quarters

1. In a food processor, combine all the ingredients except the chicken and pulse, scraping down frequently, until the paste is finely pureed.

2. Rub 6 tablespoons of the jerk paste into the chicken pieces and refrigerate overnight before cooking.

3. Fire up your grill to medium-low. Push the coals to one side of the grill and lay the chicken, skin side down, on the other side. Close the lid and cook the chicken for 25 minutes. Then flip the meat and grill until it's cooked through, 30 to 45 minutes more. (If the juices run clear when the chicken is pierced, it's done.) To infuse jerk with even more sweet, spicy flavor, add a handful of soaked pimento wood chips to the lit coals.

MAKES 6 SERVINGS · PER SERVING **776** CALORIES // **55 G** FAT // **950 MG** SODIUM // **2 G** CARBOHYDRATES // **1 G** DIETARY FIBER // **65 G** PROTEIN

SUMMER CORN

Boil corn, and you leach out valuable flavor. Cook your corn on the grill, husks intact, and you roast the kernels, concentrating their sweetness and adding a nice hit of smoke. Finish the corn Mexican-style: a squirt of lime mayo, a dusting of chili powder, and a scattering of Parmesan.

4	ears of corn
2	tablespoons mayonnaise
	Juice of 1 lime
1	teaspoon chili powder
2	tablespoons finely grated Parmesan cheese

1. Fire up a charcoal or gas grill to medium-high. Peel back the husks and remove the silk, and then re-cover the ears with the husks and soak them in cold water for 10 minutes.

2. In a small bowl, stir the mayo and lime juice together.

3. Place the ears on the grill and cook for 15 minutes, turning so the husks don't burn. Now pull back the husks and grill the ears for another 5 to 10 minutes, until the corn is lightly charred.

4. Paint the ears with a sheen of the lime mayo and dust them with the chili powder and cheese.

MAKES 4 SERVINGS · PER SERVING 154 CALORIES // 9 G FAT // 83 MG SODIUM // 19 G CARBOHYDRATES // 2 G DIETARY FIBER // 5 G PROTEIN

WATERMELON SALAD
with WARM BASIL OIL

Nothing's more refreshing on a hot summer day than biting into a sweet, juicy slice of ripe watermelon. And nothing goes better with watermelon than basil. Don't believe us? Try this simple recipe straight up, or chopped up to create a cool summertime salsa.

⅓ cup extra-virgin olive oil

⅓ cup packed basil leaves

12 thin watermelon wedges, rind removed

Thinly sliced red onion

Salt and ground black pepper

1. Heat the oil in a small saucepan. Stir in the basil, then immediately puree the mixture in a blender.

2. Arrange the watermelon wedges on 4 salad plates. Top with a little thinly sliced red onion, drizzle with 1 teaspoon of the warm basil oil, and season with salt and pepper to taste. Serve immediately.

MAKES 4 SERVINGS · PER SERVING 126 CALORIES // 5 G FAT // 158 MG SODIUM // 22 G CARBOHYDRATES // 1.5 G DIETARY FIBER // 2 G PROTEIN

BACKYARD BBQ

MEMPHIS BAKED BEANS

A few cans of baked beans isn't where this classic side dish ends—it's where it begins. At Central BBQ in Memphis, fresh vegetables and spices amp up the flavor.

3	cans (28 ounces each) baked beans (any brand)
1	onion, diced
½	red bell pepper, chopped
½	green bell pepper, chopped
½	cup yellow mustard
½	cup BBQ sauce (store-bought or homemade)
¼	cup light brown sugar
1	tablespoon minced garlic
1	tablespoon chili powder
1½	teaspoons cayenne pepper
¼	teaspoon white pepper

Preheat the oven to 275°F. In a large bowl, combine all the ingredients and pour everything into a 2-quart baking dish. Bake until the vegetables are tender and the flavors have blended, about 1 hour 30 minutes.

MAKES 8 SERVINGS · PER SERVING 393 CALORIES // 6 G FAT // 1,612 MG SODIUM // 77 G CARBOHYDRATES // 18 G DIETARY FIBER // 17 G PROTEIN

COOKOUT COLESLAW

Crisp, fresh, and sweet, coleslaw is the perfect crunchy accompaniment to rich and savory barbecue. Master this go-to recipe, then, like your barbecue sauce, experiment with different riffs to create your signature slaw. Barbecue bonus: The cabbage foundation of this side is loaded with fiber and vitamin C. A member of the famed Cruciferae (meaning "cross-bearing") plant family, cabbage is believed to contain powerful cancer-fighting properties.

2	tablespoons Dijon mustard
2	tablespoons mayonnaise
2	tablespoons vinegar (red wine, white wine, or cider)
2	tablespoons canola oil
	Salt and black pepper to taste
½	head green cabbage, very thinly sliced
½	head red cabbage, very thinly sliced
3	carrots, cut into thin strips
	Pickled jalapeños (optional)

1. Mix the mustard, mayonnaise, and vinegar in a bowl. Slowly whisk in the oil. Season with salt and pepper.

2. Combine the cabbages, carrots, jalapeños (if using), and dressing in a large bowl. Toss so that everything is evenly coated and season with more salt and pepper.

MAKES 6 SERVINGS · PER SERVING 142 CALORIES // 9 G FAT // 248 MG SODIUM // 15 G CARBOHYDRATES // 5 G DIETARY FIBER // 2 G PROTEIN

POTATO SALAD *with* ARUGULA *and* BACON

It starts with fingerling potatoes that are creamy enough when cooked to forgo an additional dollop or eight of mayonnaise. Mustard and vinegar add an acidic punch; and bacon, well, makes just about anything better, right? This dish comes courtesy of Brian Moyers, executive chef of BLT Steak in Los Angeles, California.

1	pound fingerling potatoes
	Dash of salt
½	tablespoon Dijon mustard
2	tablespoons red wine vinegar
2	tablespoons sherry vinegar
½	cup olive oil
1	tablespoon chopped fresh tarragon
4	slices thick-cut bacon, cooked and crumbled
½	rib celery, finely chopped
⅓	cup thinly sliced onion
	Salt and ground black pepper
2	cups arugula

1. Place the potatoes in a medium pot with a dash of salt. Cover with cold water, bring to a simmer, and cook the potatoes until they're fork-tender, about 10 minutes. Drain and let cool, and then halve each potato lengthwise and place in a large bowl.

2. In a small bowl, whisk together the mustard, red wine vinegar, and sherry vinegar. Gradually whisk in the olive oil. Stir in the tarragon.

3. Add the vinaigrette to the potatoes along with bacon, celery, and onion. Season with salt and pepper to taste. Refrigerate for up to 1 hour. Before serving, toss with 2 cups of arugula.

MAKES 4 SERVINGS · PER SERVING 252 CALORIES // 20 G FAT // 238 MG SODIUM // 13 G CARBOHYDRATES // 2 G DIETARY FIBER // 4 G PROTEIN

KEEP YOUR GRILLING HEALTHY
Techniques and Tips for a Better-for-You Meal

Life-threatening disease is the last thing one thinks about when sparking up the grill for a cookout. But some research suggests that eating charred meat regularly may increase cancer risk. Keep your diners safe from potential carcinogens by choosing lean cuts of meat, trimming excess fat, and avoiding charring your dinner hockey-puck black.

MARINATE TO PROTECT FROM CARCINOGENS

Before you cook, coat. Kansas State University scientists have discovered that commercial marinades reduce heterocyclic amines (HCAs)—suspected carcinogenic compounds produced by cooking meats at high temperatures—by an average of 71 percent. They believe this may be due to antioxidants in the herbs and spices that stop free-radical reactions from forming during the cooking process. Try the researchers' Caribbean beef marinade, which managed to score an 88 percent HCA reduction. Mix ¼ teaspoon each of salt, cayenne pepper, and black pepper with ½ teaspoon each of sugar, thyme, allspice, rosemary, and chives. Blend this with 2 ounces of water and 2 tablespoons each of olive oil and vinegar. For the best flavor infusion, marinate red meat overnight in the refrigerator.

DON'T OVERCOOK BURGERS

Don't burn that burger. A study in *PLOS ONE* reports that eating well-done ground beef may raise your risk of developing prostate cancer. The researchers noted a 50 percent higher risk among consumers of well-done beef than among people who ate rare to medium beef. Cooking meat "well" can create chemical compounds that have been linked to cancer, according to the study's lead author, John Witte, Ph.D., a professor at the University of California at San Francisco.

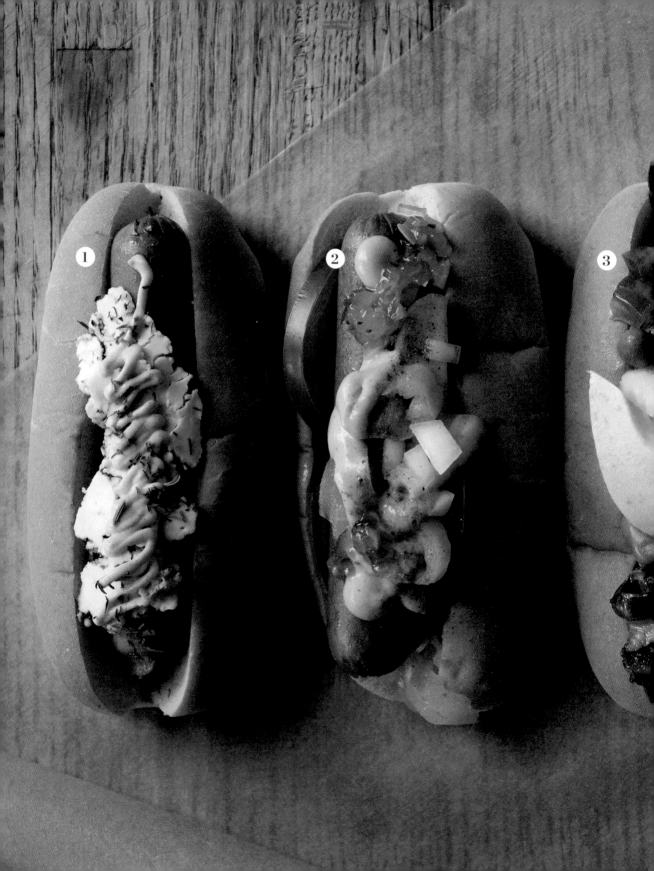

It's all about the toppings, says Doug Sohn, owner of Hot Doug's in Chicago, Illinois. Pile on . . .

1 THE FRENCHIE

Dijon mustard + blue cheese + a sprinkling of herbes de Provence

2 THE CHICAGOAN

Chopped onion + sliced tomato + yellow mustard + sweet relish + dill pickle spear + sport peppers + dash of celery salt

3 THE SONORAN

Avocado slices + mayo + chopped tomatoes + strip of crisp bacon + chopped onion + canned pinto beans

4 THE OLYMPIAN

Spinach sautéed with chopped garlic in olive oil + a brushing of Greek yogurt + a squeeze of lemon

FRIED-ONION *and* CHEDDAR BURGERS

This recipe, developed by grill master Adam Perry Lang, employs a cast-iron skillet right on the grill, allowing you to cook thinly sliced ingredients, such as sliced onions, to smoky perfection, without losing any to the flames below. The result: less mess, more flavor.

¼ cup cold water

2½ pounds ground beef (80% lean)

2 tablespoons unsalted butter

6 small to medium sweet white onions, thinly sliced

Kosher salt and ground black pepper

2 tablespoons canola oil

2 tablespoons chopped fresh flat-leaf parsley

6 thin slices cheddar cheese

6 soft hamburger buns, split and toasted

1. Set the cast-iron skillet on the grill grate and heat the grill to medium-high. In a bowl, mix the cold water into the ground beef and shape the beef into 6 patties, ¾" to 1" thick.

2. Melt 1 tablespoon of the butter in the skillet, then add the onions and season with salt and pepper. Cook, stirring occasionally, until the onions start to brown. Push the onions to one side of the skillet.

3. Season the patties with salt and pepper and brush them with the oil. Melt the remaining 1 tablespoon butter on the empty side of the skillet and add the patties. Cook the burgers until they're well seared, 2 minutes per side, and then move them onto the grill itself. Cook them until medium-rare, flipping them halfway through, about 4 minutes total.

4. Stir the parsley into the onions and spoon the mixture onto the burgers during the last minute of cooking. Lay a slice of cheese on each one and cook until it melts. Slide the patties between the buns.

MAKES 6 · PER SERVING (1 BURGER) **817** CALORIES // **58 G** FAT // **590 MG** SODIUM // **28 G** CARBOHYDRATES // **2 G** DIETARY FIBER // **44 G** PROTEIN

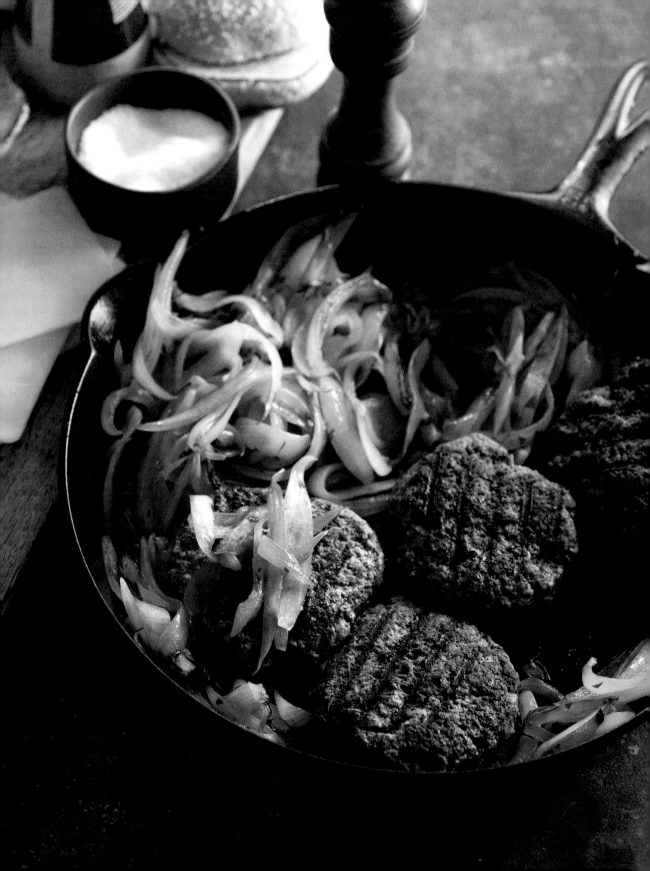

MEATLESS MEAL

A VEGGIE BURGER WORTH EATING

This recipe harnesses the rib-sticking power of black beans to serve up 6 grams of belly-filling fiber per burger.

1 COMBINE THE BASE INGREDIENTS

Quinoa and oats add plant-based protein and are especially useful for absorbing moisture and keeping the consistency manageable.

⅔ cup quinoa, cooked
(if you can find black quinoa, your patty will look more like beef)

1¾ cup canned black beans, rinsed and drained

⅔ cup rolled oats
(not quick-cooking)

2 ASSEMBLE YOUR FLAVORINGS

Now it's time to flavor your base with a few ingredients that fit within an overall theme. Mix in one of these flavoring combos, or experiment to create your own.

SOUTHWEST BURGER

3 tablespoons barbecue sauce

1 tablespoon Worcestershire sauce

2 tablespoons chopped pickled jalapeños

1 tablespoon smoked paprika

1 tablespoon chili powder

1 teaspoon ground cumin

CURRY BURGER

3 tablespoons mango chutney

2 tablespoons curry powder

¼ teaspoon kosher salt

ASIAN BURGER

3 tablespoons hoisin sauce

1 teaspoon ground ginger

1 teaspoon five-spice powder

3 PREP THE BURGER MIXTURE

Blend your ingredients in a food processor or blender, stopping as needed to scrape the sides, until the mixture is moist but holds together. If it's too thin, add more dry ingredients; if it's too thick, add more liquid flavoring.

4 PRESS INTO PATTIES AND SEAR

Set a nonstick skillet over medium heat and add 1 tablespoon of olive oil. Transfer the bean mixture to a bowl and wet your hands. Scoop out the bean mixture and press into 6 bun-size patties. Slip them carefully into the hot pan, one at a time, until the pan is full but not crowded. Cook the patties until they acquire a crispy crust, about 4 minutes on each side.

MAKES 4 · PER SERVING (1 BURGER) **441** CALORIES // **20 G** FAT // **860 MG** SODIUM // **28 G** CARBOHYDRATES // **3 G** DIETARY FIBER // **38 G** PROTEIN

5 BRING ON THE TOPPINGS

There's no need to overthrow the holy trinity of lettuce, tomato, and onion, but the inspired burger chef may want to switch it up. Layer on big flavor with these under-the-radar toppings.

PICKLED JALAPEÑOS

They deliver the acidic bite of red onion but with the added perk of capsaicin. Buy the presliced kind for no-prep heat.

ROASTED RED PEPPERS

Red peppers are not only appealing to the eye but also have more than twice the vitamin E and 10 times the vitamin A of green peppers. The jarred roasted kind work great—just blot off any excess liquid.

AVOCADO

There's relatively little fat in beans or grains, but by adding avocado you'll restore the rich mouthfeel you've come to expect from a burger. To identify a ripe, creamy avocado, give it a gentle squeeze; it should yield slightly.

PINEAPPLE

Drop full rings onto a grill or grill pan and give them a few minutes on each side for crispy, caramelized stripes. Canned rings work fine, but pat them dry with a paper towel first.

RYAN FARR'S SPICY LAMB BURGER *with* SCALLIONS

Farr is a butcher for 4505 Meats in San Francisco, California. He serves up these nontraditional burgers at the Ferry Building Marketplace.

1 pound lamb sirloin, ground

½ teaspoon ground coriander

½ teaspoon ground black pepper

1 teaspoon salt

1½ tablespoons mayonnaise

1½ tablespoons sour cream

1 tablespoon milk

1 tablespoon harissa paste (find it in the international section of the supermarket)

4 slices Gruyère cheese

4 potato buns, split and toasted

⅓ cup chopped scallions

1. Sprinkle the lamb with the coriander, pepper, and 1 teaspoon of the salt; fold until blended, about 1 minute. Divide the meat into quarters and form into ½" patties. Refrigerate 15 minutes.

2. In a bowl, combine the mayo, sour cream, milk, harissa, and a dash of salt. Set aside.

3. On a hot, well-oiled grill or cast-iron pan set on medium high, cook the patties until seared, 1 to 1½ minutes. Flip them and top each with Gruyère. Cook until medium-rare, 1 minute more.

4. Place the burgers on the bottom part of the buns. Slather the cut sides of the top buns with the sauce and sprinkle with scallions. Close the buns and serve.

MAKES 4 · PER SERVING (1 BURGER) 441 CALORIES // 20 G FAT // 860 MG SODIUM // 28 G CARBOHYDRATES // 3 G DIETARY FIBER // 38 G PROTEIN

○ GRIND YOUR OWN BURGER MEAT

Freshly ground meat makes mind-blowing burgers. No grinder? Try our food processor method.

1 Cut the meat into 1½" cubes and place them, along with the blade and bucket of a food processor, onto a baking sheet. Pop everything into the freezer until the cubes are slightly frozen around the edges.

2 Put the cold meat into the cold food processor. Pulse until it's chopped but still slightly chunky. Transfer it to a bowl and refrigerate until you're ready to use it.

GRILLED SOY-LEMON CHICKEN UNDER A BRICK

Topping the split bird with a brick presses down the legs and breasts onto the grill grates, so they reach tender, juicy doneness at the same time, says Chris Lily, chef and partner at Big Bob Gibson's Bar-B-Q in Decatur, Alabama. Wrap with foil first. The brick, that is.

½	cup soy sauce
¼	cup lemon juice
4	tablespoons unsalted butter, melted
¾	teaspoon ground black pepper
¾	teaspoon garlic powder
½	teaspoon ground ginger
½	teaspoon sugar
1	whole chicken (3 to 3½ pounds), split in half, backbone removed

1. In a bowl, whisk together all the ingredients except the chicken. Reserve ⅓ cup of the marinade for basting; pour the rest into a resealable plastic bag. Add the chicken, turning to coat. Seal the bag and refrigerate for at least 30 minutes (or up to overnight).

2. When you're ready to cook, wrap two bricks separately in doubled heavy-duty foil. Preheat the grill to medium low.

3. Place the chicken halves on the grill, skin side down. Place a brick over each half, cover the grill, and cook until their internal temperature reaches 165°F, 40 to 45 minutes, turning and basting them halfway through.

MAKES 4 SERVINGS · PER SERVING **637** CALORIES // **46 G** FAT // **1,297 MG** SODIUM // **3 G** CARBOHYDRATES // **0 G** DIETARY FIBER // **51 G** PROTEIN

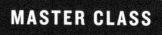

KEBABS

In an age of microwave ovens and induction cooktops, few foods feel more primal and effortless than meat on a stick. Skewer some protein and throw it on the grill, and you've created a quick summer meal. But give kebabs a bit more attention—a homemade marinade, some well-chosen add-ons, a sauce alongside—and you can create the best kebabs on the block.

You have a smorgasbord of options to explore here: Stick to the classics by marinating lamb in yogurt with Indian spices and pairing it with a classic combo of zucchini, peppers, and onion. Soak beef in a teriyaki marinade and skewer it alongside Japanese-style accents, such as scallions and pickled ginger. Or try citrusy shrimp with the Italian triumvirate of prosciutto, tomato, and basil. When it comes to meat on a stick, you're in charge of your own delicious destiny.

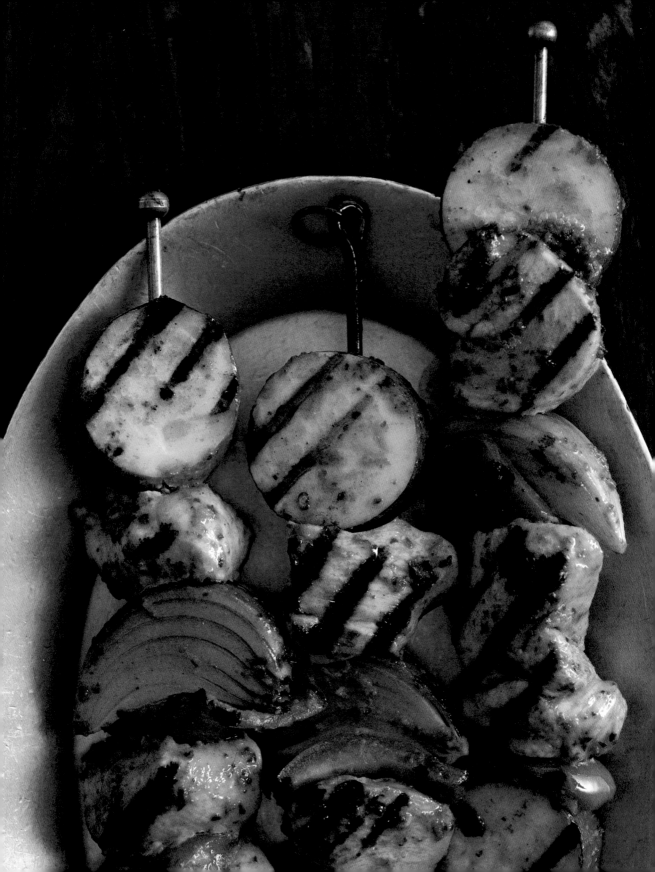

1 PICK YOUR PROTEIN

For 4 servings, start with 1½ pounds of meat or seafood cut into 1" chunks. Kebabs cook through quickly, so crank your grill to high for a good sear.

CHICKEN

Go with boneless, skinless breasts and/or thighs. (We're thigh folks ourselves—dark meat is more flavorful.)

Cooking Time: About 5 minutes

BEEF

Blade, flatiron, and skirt steaks have the best balance of tenderness and beefy essence.

Cooking Time: 2 to 4 minutes for medium-rare

TUNA

Think of tuna as steak of the sea. It's a perfect fish to serve rare, letting the marinade's flavors shine through.

Cooking Time: About 2 minutes for rare

2 CHOOSE YOUR MARINADE

Small chunks of protein absorb a marinade's flavor in just an hour. Reserve some marinade before you add the protein, and serve it at the table.

CURRIED YOGURT

1 cup whole-milk yogurt + 1 teaspoon curry powder + 1 teaspoon salt + ½ teaspoon ground black pepper

TERIYAKI

1 teaspoon minced garlic + 1 teaspoon minced fresh ginger + ½ cup soy sauce + 1 tablespoon sugar

SPICY MOROCCAN

In a blender, puree 1 jarred roasted red bell pepper + 3 tablespoons olive oil + 3 cloves garlic + 2 teaspoons red-pepper flakes + 1 teaspoon each of salt, ground cumin, and coriander.

3 MIX IT UP

Experiment with add-ons. Cut them into 1" pieces as needed, and then thread them onto skewers, alternating with the meat or seafood.

ZUCCHINI/RED PEPPER/ONION

This classic combo is a nod to Italy—and to summer. Skewer zucchini slices through the skin so they don't spin as you turn the kebabs.

PROSCIUTTO/ TOMATO/BASIL

Wrap a slice of prosciutto around a cherry tomato before skewering, and alternate with the meat and whole basil leaves.

OKRA/SMOKY BACON

Bacon crisps up nicely on the grill, adding a smoky note to green okra.

LAMB

Its bold flavor stands up to a spicy marinade. Pick boneless leg or rib chops for maximum tenderness.

Cooking Time: 2 to 4 minutes for medium-rare

SHRIMP

Choose large shrimp that have been peeled and deveined. You can tell shrimp are done when they're firm and pink, with a bit of char.

Cooking Time: 3 to 4 minutes

BLACK OLIVE AND CAPER

½ cup finely chopped and pitted kalamata olives + ¼ cup olive oil + ¼ cup chopped capers + 3 minced cloves garlic + 1 tablespoon lemon juice + 1 teaspoon ground black pepper

LEMON-PEPPER

⅓ cup olive oil + 1 teaspoon grated lemon zest + ¼ cup lemon juice + 2 finely chopped cloves garlic + 1 teaspoon salt + 1 teaspoon ground black pepper

GREEN BEAN/ POTATO/ MUSHROOM

These add-ons elevate kebabs to a full-blown meal. Use halved cremini mushrooms, along with baby red potatoes that have been boiled for 15 minutes and then halved.

SCALLIONS/ PICKLED GINGER

These ingredients add instant sweet and savory Asian flavors. Use them with steak for a version of the Japanese beef dish *negimaki;* with tuna, the result is almost like grilled sushi.

4 THE FINISHING TOUCH

EASY LEMON AIOLI

This flavorful French mayonnaise adds a creamy kick to kebabs. To make it in minutes, use a shortcut: store-bought mayo.

Whisk together ½ cup olive-oil mayonnaise with 1 finely chopped clove garlic, 1 teaspoon grated lemon zest, and 2 teaspoons lemon juice. Season with a pinch of salt and pepper.

CILANTRO CHIMICHURRI

This simple South American sauce adds freshness to grilled meats.

In a food processor, combine 1 cup cilantro leaves, ½ cup olive oil, ⅓ cup lime juice, 2 chopped cloves garlic, and ½ teaspoon each of red-pepper flakes and salt. Pulse the ingredients until they're finely chopped.

SPICY CHILI SAUCE

Smear on this hot and sweet sauce during grilling for an extra layer of heat, or use it for dipping at the table. (Have a beer nearby to extinguish the chili flames.)

To make it, stir together ⅓ cup Asian chili sauce and ⅓ cup maple syrup, and mix in 2 finely chopped scallions.

SMOKE JOINT PRIME RIB

You haven't tasted prime rib until you've experienced it pulled out of a smoker. This recipe, developed by Craig Samuel of Smoke Joint in Brooklyn, New York, takes an afternoon to cook, but we promise this will be some of the best meat you'll ever eat. Round up some friends, crack some beers, and enjoy.

1½ cups dark brown sugar

½ cup kosher salt

½ cup butcher-grind black pepper (spicebarn.com) or coarsely ground black pepper

3 tablespoons sweet paprika

1 tablespoon smoked paprika or chile powder

1 teaspoon cayenne pepper

1 teaspoon garlic powder

½ teaspoon onion powder

½ teaspoon mustard powder

1 boneless rib eye roast (10 to 14 pounds)

1–3 hickory chunks or 2 cups chips

1. In a large bowl, combine ½ cup of the brown sugar, the salt, black pepper, paprikas, cayenne, garlic powder, onion powder, and mustard powder. Generously coat the roast with ⅓ of the mixture, but don't rub it in. (Reserve the rest for another day—it works great on any steak or pork, for roasting or for grilling.) Loosely cover the roast and refrigerate it for at least 4 hours or up to overnight.

2. An hour before cooking, remove the meat from the fridge and let it sit at room temperature. Pat the roast dry with a paper towel, taking care not to loosen the spices. Then press the remaining 1 cup brown sugar onto all sides of the roast.

3. Soak the wood for 20 minutes, then drain. Fire up the barbecue for indirect heat. Fill a large aluminum foil pan with ⅛" of water. Remove the grill grates, place the pan in the center of the grill (away from the coals), and replace the grates.

4. Cook the roast at 250°F until a meat thermometer in the thickest part of the meat registers 130°F for rare, 3½ to 4 hours.

5. Let the meat rest for 30 minutes before carving, and serve it with the cooking juices from the foil pan.

MAKES 15 SERVINGS · PER SERVING 559 CALORIES // 24 G FAT // 557 MG SODIUM // 15 G CARBOHYDRATES // 0 G DIETARY FIBER // 67 G PROTEIN

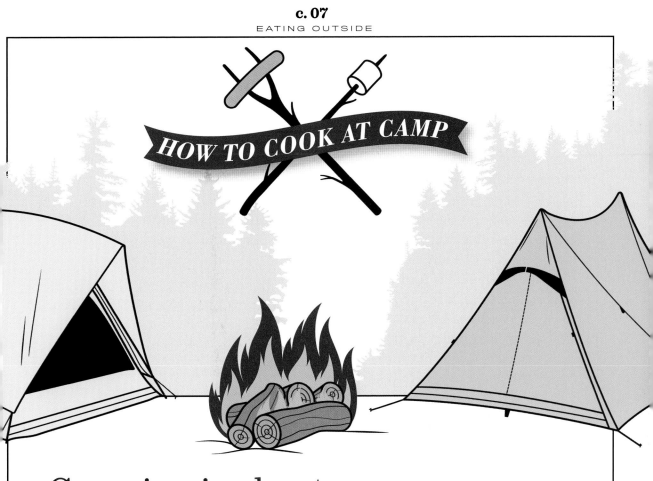

HOW TO COOK AT CAMP

Camping is about making a temporary home in the permanent home of bears, raccoons, and fire ants. Once the tent is up and you've figured out the latrine situation, the rest is about the cooking. You'll enjoy camping a lot more if you get the food right. That means being prepared: planning out your meals and having the right ingredients on hand. You can go all-out fancy, but remember, you're still eating in the dirt. So keep things simple and hearty.

HOW TO COOK AT CAMP

CAVEMAN POTATOES AND ROASTED CORN

Get a good hardwood fire going. Allow the fire to burn down to a bed of red-hot coals. Take a stick and rake the coals into a mound. Use the stick to dig a hole a little deeper than the thickness of your potatoes. (If you think of it, dig the hole before you build the fire.) Drop the potatoes into the hole and cover with ½" of dirt. Push the hot coals over them. Now add some kindling to build up the fire again. You're going to bake those spuds for about an hour, so add some 2"-diameter logs to the fire to keep it going. After 30 minutes, let the fire return to coals. Meanwhile, peel the husks down to the bottom of your ears of corn but without ripping them off. Pull out the silk, and then close up the husks. Soak the ears in water for a few minutes, then place them directly on the glowing coals. Turn occasionally as they roast for 15 minutes. They should be roasted nicely by the time you're ready to dig your baked potatoes out of the dirt. Hope you remembered the butter and Old Bay.

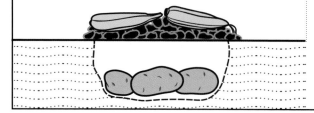

STICK FISH

This works best for long, narrow fish like trout and pickerel, but can be employed for bass and panfish, too. Gut and clean your fish as soon as you can after catching and cook ASAP if you can't ice down the fish to preserve the flavor.

Build a good fire and allow to burn down to small flames. Cut a green switch and use your knife to shave one end into a point.

Rub the cavity of the fish with butter or olive oil and sprinkle with salt and pepper. Pierce the skin side of the tail end of the fish with the pointed stick and work the stick through, guiding it up through the cavity, and poke it through the thicker flesh at the top to secure.

Using heavy rocks, support the fish stick over the flames. Lower it closer to the coals as the fire dies down. (Another option is to lay the fish-on-a-stick right on the bed of glowing embers and turn halfway through cooking.)

When done, hold the stick to eat the fish as if it was a corndog.

HOW TO EAT A PINE TREE

Let's say you're lost in the wilderness for several days without a Snickers bar. Or maybe a bear got into your cooler and made off with your beef bourguignon and you don't feel like getting into the car for McDonald's. It's nice to know how to forage for a meal so you won't go hungry in the woods. Here are some wild edibles to gnaw on.*

GREENS

DANDELION, PURSLANE, CHICORY, WATERCRESS

Eat them raw or boil them tender. Clip the new shoots off the common milkweed plant and boil until tender. Eat as you would asparagus.

TUBERS

THE ROOTS OF CATTAIL PLANTS, ARROWHEAD, WILD ONION, AND DAY LILY

Boil them or roast on hot coals. Wrap them in large green leaves soaked in water to steam first. Cattail on the cob: Boil the young green flower spikes of cattail plants and eat them like corn on the cob.

BERRIES

BLUEBERRIES, RASPBERRIES, HUCKLEBERRIES, BLACKBERRIES, BEACH PLUM, AND WILD GRAPE

Eat as is or use to flavor water or make into desserts.

NUTS

CHESTNUT, HICKORY, BLACK WALNUT, HAZELNUT

Crack 'em and eat 'em or roast them in hot coals.

OAKS AND PINES

Peel off the brown outer bark of oak trees, pine trees, and beechwood trees to get at the thin "inner skin" in between. Peel this and eat it raw. Tastes like…well, a tree.

But it's nutritious. Pine needles are edible and can be used for tea. Baby pinecones and the seeds from mature cones are edible, too.

BEVERAGES

Steep the leaves of spearmint or peppermint in boiling water for hot tea. Take the red clusters of staghorn sumac and steep them in water to make a pink "lemonade." Sweeten with sugar and lemons if you have 'em.

* For safety, consult an illustrated field guide to edible plants before dining on the bounty of the outdoors.

HOW TO COOK AT CAMP

BISCUITS ON A GREEN STICK

Cut one or two green branches about 2 feet long and 1½" in diameter. Leave the bumps and nubs where the smaller branches were; you might even score the branch with your knife so the dough will hold better on it. Mix your dough from water and Bisquick or another biscuit flour and pat it into long 2"-wide strips. Take a strip and wrap it around the green stick— the part that will hover over the coals.
(The bottom end will go into the dirt or be held at an angle with rocks.)
Be sure to leave some space between the turns of the dough so it doesn't touch. Angle the dough spit over your coals and rotate occasionally to bake evenly.

BURGER TENTS

Place a large piece of heavy-duty aluminum foil on a flat surface. Put 1 hamburger patty or a hamburger's worth of ground beef on the foil and add sliced carrots, celery, potatoes, onions, a teaspoon of Montreal steak seasoning, and 3 tablespoons of water.
Fold over the foil to seal the edges. Poke the tines of a fork in the top of the foil to allow steam to escape. Place the foil packet on the hot campfire coals and cook for 20 to 30 minutes.
Cleanup is easy because your foil pouch is your plate. Instead of ground beef, try this with chunks of beef or chicken breast or fish. Reduce cooking time if using fish.

COWBOY COFFEE

Add a quart of fresh water to an enamel or metal coffeepot. Set it over the flame or on coals to boil. When you've got a roiling boil, remove the pot and add ¾ cup of ground coffee (or a bit more if you like it stronger). Return the pot to a roiling boil for 1 minute, then remove the pot again and set it in the dirt for 5 minutes to allow the grounds to sink. Pour the coffee carefully to avoid stirring up the grounds. Some folks think getting grounds in their teeth is part of the charm of cowboy coffee, and they even like the nutty crunch. If you're more of a dude than a ranch hand, you can pour the coffee through a bandanna to screen out the grounds.

CAMPFIRE FISH

Outdoor cooking should be more than just charred hot dogs, says Johan Svensson, executive chef of Aquavit in New York City and a former soldier in the Swedish army. "If you're cooking with pots, pans, and gas, there will be no quintessential smoky flavor added," he says. That's chef parlance for boring. Fish pairs well with flame.

1	trout (3 to 4 pounds), gutted
	Salt and ground black pepper
1	onion, thinly sliced
1	tomato, thinly sliced
1	sprig thyme or pine needles, rinsed
1	lemon, halved
30"	butchers' twine, cut into thirds
1	tablespoon oil

1. With a clean, wet rag or brush, scrub a flat stone. Carefully place it in a bed of red coals or wood embers contained within a fire ring, or make the fire around the stone. Let heat for 45 minutes. (It's ready when a few drops of water pearl upon impact instead of soaking in.)

2. Season the fish inside and out with salt and pepper. Stuff the cavity with onion, tomato, and thyme or pine needles, and then add the juice of half a lemon. Cut the rest of the lemon into segments and place them in the cavity.

3. Tie the fish with twine and rub it with the oil to crisp the skin and prevent sticking. Use a large spatula or tongs to place it on the stone.

4. Cook until the flesh flakes fairly easily, 6 to 8 minutes a side.

MAKES 2 SERVINGS · PER SERVING 574 CALORIES // 25 G FAT // 271 MG SODIUM // 14 G CARBOHYDRATES // 4 G DIETARY FIBER // 73 G PROTEIN

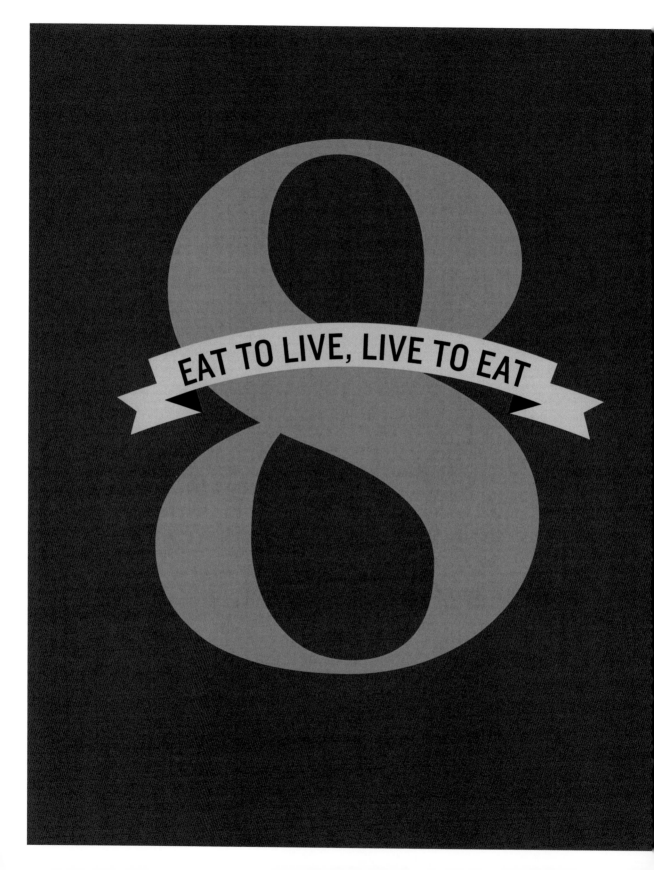

EAT TO LIVE, LIVE TO EAT

DATE NIGHT

As long as the food is good and you make the evening all about her, you'll earn four stars, chef.

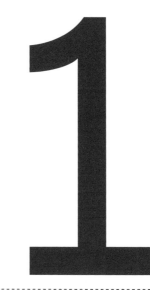

p. 216   GUY **MH** GOURMET   c. 08

COOKING *for* HER

In dating, as in life, you never want them to see you sweat. And that goes double for cooking. There's no point in laboring over a recipe you've never tried, neglecting her because you're too stressed over your crème brûlée. Keep it simple, make it look easy, and she'll come back for more.

RULE Nº

1

DEMO SOME FORWARD THINKING

WOMEN NOTICE SHOES. (Keep yours shined.) Women also notice effort. So demonstrate the fact that you've planned this dinner date by cleaning up your place, selecting a music soundtrack, and considering her tastes in food. For music, dig into your playlist and put on something unusual (or even embarrassing) that you're obsessed with, and you'll actually have something to talk about, not just listen to.

RULE Nº 2 | MAKE HER COMFORTABLE

WHEN SHE ARRIVES, have a drink and perhaps a snack ready to keep her occupied while you finish cooking. Better yet, stop what you're doing and have a drink with her; this will show that she's more important than the dinner and that the kitchen is under control. She'll probably ask, "What can I do to help?" Your first answer is "Nothing. Have a drink and relax." If she seems truly eager to assist, let her pitch in, but pick a task that's not mundane or intimidating. (Chopping parsley = fun. Scaling fish = punishment.)

RULE Nº 3 | DON'T SERVE A PLATE OF CLICHÉS

SKIP THE CHOCOLATE-dipped strawberries. Instead, start with a dish you know she likes (you'll show you've been listening), and then make the recipe your own by adding or subtracting an ingredient or changing up the presentation. Have a "signature" pasta dish you can make on autopilot? Transform it into something you haven't cooked for countless others by giving it a twist—a pinch of curry, a side of vegetables from the farmers' market. Or just stick to a simple but surprising make-ahead menu.

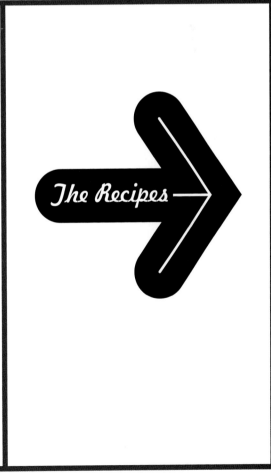

The Recipes →

SEARED SCALLOPS *with* WHITE BEANS *and* BACON

If she's a fan of scallops, serve her this dish, which elevates the subtle flavor of the mollusks with savory bacon and creamy white beans. Plus, it takes relatively little time out of your evening. What you two choose to do with that extra time is up to you.

---

1   slice bacon, chopped into small pieces

¼   red onion, minced

1   clove garlic, minced

1⅓   cups white beans (from a 15-ounce can), rinsed and drained

2   cups baby spinach

½   pound large sea scallops

Salt and ground black pepper

1   tablespoon butter

Juice of ½ lemon

1. Cook the bacon in a medium saucepan over low heat until it begins to crisp. Pour off some of the bacon fat and add the onion and garlic. Cook until the onion is soft and translucent, 2 to 3 minutes. Add the beans and spinach and cook until the beans are hot and the spinach is wilted. Keep warm.

2. Heat a large cast-iron skillet or sauté pan over medium-high heat. Blot the scallops dry with a paper towel and season them on both sides with salt and pepper to taste. Add the butter to the pan. After it melts, add the scallops. Sear them on each side until they're deeply caramelized.

3. Before serving, add the lemon juice to the beans, along with some salt and pepper. Divide the beans between 2 warm bowls or plates and top with the scallops.

MAKES 2 SERVINGS · PER SERVING **284** CALORIES // **7 G** FAT // **400 MG** SODIUM // **28 G** CARBOHYDRATES // **7 G** DIETARY FIBER // **28 G** PROTEIN

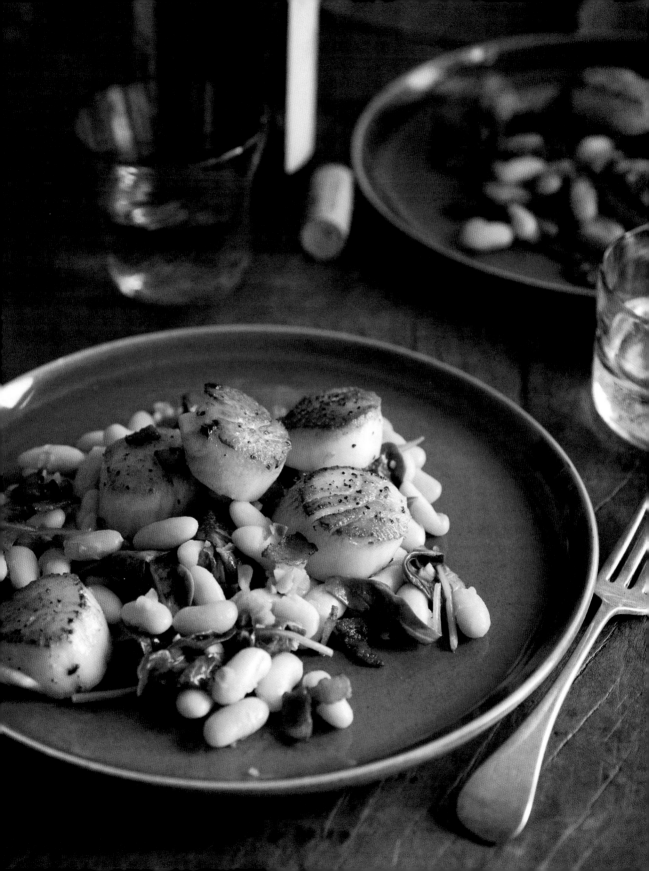

CRAB CAKES

This spin on crab cakes comes from Eric Ripert, executive chef of one of New York City's greatest restaurants, Le Bernardin. The secret to this recipe, he swears, is the perfect heat your toaster oven provides to crisp the cakes just right. Who knew the device you used to heat up your pizza bagels in college could help you win her heart? Serve it as an appetizer or as a main course with a few simple sides such as steamed spinach with a squeeze of lemon juice and drizzle of olive oil.

8	ounces jumbo lump crabmeat
¼	cup sour cream
1	teaspoon Dijon mustard
1	teaspoon Worcestershire sauce
1	teaspoon Old Bay seasoning
2	teaspoons lemon juice
¼	cup panko bread crumbs, plus extra for topping
	Fine sea salt and ground white pepper to taste

Remove the toaster oven tray and turn the heat to 425°F. In a bowl, combine all the ingredients and gently stir to evenly coat the crabmeat, being careful not to break it up too much. Place two 3½" ring molds on the tray. Divide the crab mixture between them, sprinkle on more panko, and then gently remove the molds. Bake the crab cakes until the tops are golden brown, 8 to 10 minutes.

MAKES 2 SERVINGS · PER SERVING 182 CALORIES // 6 G FAT // 907 MG SODIUM // 10 G CARBOHYDRATES // 0 G DIETARY FIBER // 21 G PROTEIN

✚ KITCHEN EMT ✚
DON'T BUTTER YOUR BURN

If you burn your hand picking up a hot pot, run cold water over the injury. Lots of cold water. The coolness acts as a painkiller and stops the burn from spreading through your tissue. For that reason, leave the butter for your bread; grandma's folk remedy only holds in the heat you want to get rid of. If hot oil or grease splatters you, same deal: lots of cold water. But if the grease saturated your clothing and the fabric is sticking to your skin, don't try to remove it. Douse with lots of cold water, then go to a doctor.

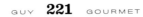

WARM GOAT CHEESE SALAD
with FRIED EGG

Serve your lady a salad appetizer out of a bag with some bottled dressing and she's going to question your cooking skills—and your enthusiasm. Follow this simple recipe, courtesy of James Boyce, chef of Cotton Row in Huntsville, Alabama, to show her she's worth the extra effort. To save time, make the dressing and bread the goat cheese and chill it before she arrives. That way, when it's game time, all you have to do is sear the goat cheese, fry the eggs, and toss the salad.

	Juice of ½ lemon
1	teaspoon grainy mustard
1	teaspoon chopped capers
2½	tablespoons olive oil
	Salt and ground black pepper
1½	tablespoons all-purpose flour
1	egg, beaten with splash of milk
¼	cup unseasoned dry bread crumbs
½	log fresh goat cheese (4 ounces), cut into 8 rounds
2	eggs
2	cups watercress or other leafy green

1. In a large bowl, whisk together the lemon juice, mustard, capers, and 1½ tablespoons of the oil. Season with salt and pepper to taste and set aside.

2. In three separate shallow bowls, place the flour, egg mixture, and bread crumbs. Coat each piece of cheese in the flour, then the egg mixture, and finally the bread crumbs, pressing firmly to make sure they adhere.

3. Heat a large nonstick skillet over medium heat. When the pan is hot, add the remaining 1 tablespoon oil and swirl it around the pan. Add the cheese rounds and cook until golden brown, about 2 minutes a side. Transfer the cheese to paper towels.

4. With the pan still over medium heat, crack in the eggs and fry until the whites solidify.

5. To serve, toss the watercress with the dressing, and top each serving with 2 rounds of goat cheese and a fried egg.

MAKES 2 SERVINGS · PER SERVING **527** CALORIES // **41 G** FAT // **607 MG** SODIUM // **17 G** CARBOHYDRATES // **1 G** DIETARY FIBER // **23 G** PROTEIN

STEAK AU POIVRE *with* ROAST POTATOES *and* GREEN BEANS

Women love steak, too—as long as you cook it nicely. This is old-school, highbrow French fare, sure to pique her palate, made in about 30 minutes. The best part? You'll love eating it, too.

½ pound fingerling potatoes, scrubbed

3 tablespoons extra-virgin olive oil

1 tablespoon finely chopped fresh rosemary

Salt and ground black pepper

2 strip steaks (6 ounces each)

2 tablespoons black peppercorns, crushed

2 tablespoons unsalted butter

½ pound haricots verts (thin French green beans)

1 shallot, finely chopped

¼ cup brandy

½ cup low-sodium beef broth

2 teaspoons green peppercorns, in brine, drained and coarsely chopped

¼ cup heavy cream

1. Preheat the oven to 400°F. On a baking sheet, toss the potatoes with 2 tablespoons of the oil, the rosemary and salt and pepper to taste. Roast until browned and fork-tender, about 25 minutes.

2. Meanwhile, coat the steaks with the crushed peppercorns. In a large skillet or stainless steel sauté pan, heat 1 tablespoon of the butter and the remaining 1 tablespoon olive oil over medium-high heat. Add the steaks to the pan and cook, without turning, until a crust has formed, 3 to 4 minutes. Flip the steaks and cook for an additional 3 to 4 minutes or medium-rare. Transfer the steaks to a plate and cover with foil to keep warm.

3. Place a vegetable steamer basket into a pot with an inch of water in it and bring to a boil. Place the haricots verts in the steamer basket, cover the pot, and steam until the beans are tender yet still firm and bright green, about 5 minutes. Remove from the heat and season with salt and pepper.

4. Melt the remaining 1 tablespoon butter in the pan you used to cook the steak over medium heat. Add the shallot and cook until soft. Stir in the brandy, scraping the bottom of the pan to get up any browned bits. Add the broth and green peppercorns, boiling until slightly reduced. Stir in the cream. Boil another 2 to 3 minutes to thicken the sauce. Spoon the sauce over the steaks and serve with the haricots verts and potatoes.

MAKES 2 SERVINGS · PER SERVING 913 CALORIES // 55 G FAT // 285 MG SODIUM // 39 G CARBOHYDRATES // 7 G DIETARY FIBER // 46 G PROTEIN

AGE YOUR STEAK AT HOME

The aging process

is what separates top-dollar steak-houses from sit-down chains. As beef ages, the longer protein chains within the muscles break down. As aging creates more of these protein fragments, the meat becomes more tender and flavorful.

Most high-end chophouses age their beef for at least 30 days, but you can tenderize your beef simply by being lazy. Just leave your steaks in their packaging in the refrigerator for 5 days before cooking. They'll change color but won't go bad.

CREATE YOUR OWN MARINADE

ONE PART ACID
Start with an acid to add bite to the marinade. You can use lemon juice, white wine vinegar, or balsamic vinegar.

ONE PART OIL
To balance the taste, carry the flavor, and contribute a subtle nuttiness, try olive oil, canola oil, or grapeseed oil.

ADD SOME FLAVOR
Shallots, ginger, and herbs (chives, parsley) add tang. Use red-pepper flakes for a spicier edge.

FINISH IT OFF
Season the steak with kosher salt and freshly ground black pepper, both of which transfer the seasoning to the meat. Then soak your steak for 2 to 12 hours. (Longer is better.)

SEA BASS *with* ASPARAGUS

Sea bass carries a pleasant, buttery taste that isn't too fishy. Pair it with fresh asparagus in the spring or summer, or broccoli florets when the weather cools down.

2   fillets (6 ounces each) sea bass, halibut, or another firm white fish

6   asparagus spears

2   ounces shiitake mushrooms, stems discarded

1½   teaspoons grated fresh ginger

1   tablespoon low-sodium soy sauce

1   tablespoon mirin (sweetened rice wine) or sake

     Salt and ground black pepper

1. Preheat the oven to 400°F. Tear off two 12" squares of foil. Lay the foil pieces on a counter and place a fillet in the middle of each one. Scatter the asparagus, mushrooms, and ginger on top of the fish.

2. Drizzle each fillet with soy sauce and mirin and season with a small pinch of salt and black pepper.

3. Fold the foil over the ingredients and crimp the edges to seal. Place the packets on a large baking sheet and bake until the fish flakes easily, 20 to 25 minutes, depending on the thickness of the fillets.

MAKES 2 SERVINGS · PER SERVING **253** CALORIES // **5 G** FAT // **457 MG** SODIUM // **7 G** CARBOHYDRATES // **2 G** DIETARY FIBER // **42 G** PROTEIN

CHIPOTLE SWEET POTATO FONDUE

This sexy-as-hell recipe from Peggy Fallon, author of *Great Party Fondues*, gives your date a reason to indulge.

1½   teaspoons unsalted butter

½   medium onion, chopped

¾   pound sweet potatoes, peeled and coarsely chopped

1¾   cups chicken broth

½   teaspoon canned chipotle peppers in adobo sauce

¼   cup sour cream, plus more for serving

Juice of ½ lime

Sea salt

1 or 2 tablespoons chopped fresh cilantro (optional)

1. Melt the butter in a large saucepan over medium heat. Add the onion and cook to soften, 3 to 5 minutes. Add the sweet potatoes and broth. Cover and simmer until the potatoes are tender, about 20 minutes. Cool slightly.

2. Puree the sweet potatoes (and broth) with the chipotle pepper in a blender until smooth. Return them to the saucepan and whisk in ¼ cup sour cream and the lime juice. (Add more broth or water if it's too thick.) Add salt to taste and cook over medium-low heat for 5 minutes.

3. Transfer the mixture to a fondue pot. Garnish with cilantro and more sour cream, if desired. Adjust the heat under the pot so your fondue is warm, not boiling. Serve with cooked shrimp, hearty artisan bread, and assorted crudités. Don't eat directly off the poking fork, though—you risk burning your lips.

MAKES 2 ENTRÉE SERVINGS · PER SERVING **254** CALORIES // **10 G** FAT // **1,021 MG** SODIUM // **35 G** CARBOHYDRATES // **5 G** DIETARY FIBER // **5 G** PROTEIN

ORZOTTO *with* BURST TOMATOES

Risotto, made with short-grain rice, is often tricky. This mistake-proof dish uses rice-shaped pasta instead. Make it an hour or two ahead, and then gently reheat.

4	tablespoons extra-virgin olive oil
1	pint cherry tomatoes
1	clove garlic, thinly sliced
10	basil leaves, plus more for serving
	Salt
2	cups chicken or vegetable broth
2	cups water
¼	cup finely chopped onion
1	cup orzo pasta
¼	cup white wine
¼	cup grated Parmesan cheese, plus more for serving
	Ground black pepper

1. Heat 2 tablespoons of the oil in a skillet over medium-high heat. Add the tomatoes and cook, tossing occasionally, until they begin to burst and collapse, about 5 minutes. Add the garlic and cook until fragrant, about 3 minutes. Press the tomatoes with a spoon until they all pop and release some of their juice; stir the sauce together. Stack the basil leaves and roll them up like a cigar. Thinly slice the basil crosswise and toss it into the tomatoes. Season with salt to taste, then cover to keep warm.

2. In a saucepan, bring the broth and water to a simmer.

3. In another skillet, heat the remaining 2 tablespoons oil over medium heat. Add the onion and cook, stirring frequently, until soft, about 5 minutes. Add the orzo and cook, stirring, until lightly toasted, about 2 minutes. Add the wine and cook until evaporated.

4. Ladle in 1 cup of the hot broth and simmer, stirring constantly, until the liquid is almost absorbed. Add another ladleful, again waiting until it's nearly absorbed before adding more. Keep adding liquid in this fashion until the orzo is tender and the mixture is thickened, about 20 minutes. Stir in the tomato mixture and the Parmesan. Season to taste with salt and pepper, top with more cheese and basil, and serve.

MAKES 2 SERVINGS · PER SERVING **681** CALORIES // **33 G** FAT // **1,074 MG** SODIUM // **74 G** CARBOHYDRATES // **6 G** DIETARY FIBER // **19 G** PROTEIN

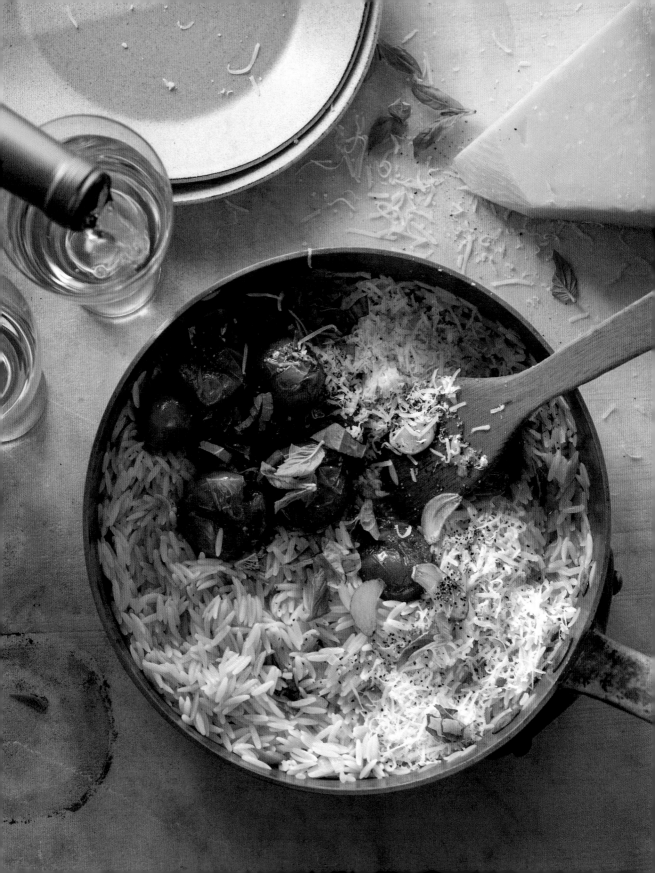

POLLO ALLA DIAVOLA

Roasting a chicken has always been a great way to score points effortlessly. This version cooks up fast—and looks amazing on a platter. Start a day ahead by marinating the bird. After you roast it, you'll make a quick pan sauce. "The chicken's great with sautéed broccoli rabe or roasted potatoes," says Nick Anderer, chef of Maialino in New York City.

3 tablespoons extra-virgin olive oil

1 teaspoon coarse salt

6 sprigs of fresh thyme

Cracked black pepper

Red-pepper flakes

1 whole chicken (3 to 4 pounds), butterflied (ask the butcher to do this, or use four leg quarters)

1 cup low-sodium chicken broth

1 cup pickling liquid from jarred hot cherry peppers, plus peppers for serving

2 tablespoons tomato sauce or puree

1. The day before you cook the chicken, combine the oil, salt, thyme, and cracked black pepper and pepper flakes to taste in a wide baking dish. Add the chicken, turning it to coat it evenly, then cover and refrigerate it overnight.

2. Half an hour before you're ready to cook, remove the chicken from the fridge. Preheat the oven to 375°F. Place a cast-iron skillet or other ovenproof pan in the preheated oven until it's medium hot, about 5 minutes.

3. Remove the pan from the oven and add the chicken, skin side down. Then add another cast-iron skillet on top of the bird to weight it down. Place the chicken in the oven to roast until it's golden brown and juices run clear when it's pierced in the hip joint, 45 to 55 minutes. Remove the chicken to a cutting board to rest, leaving the juices in the pan.

4. To make the sauce, place the pan over medium-low heat and whisk in the broth, pickling liquid, and tomato sauce, scraping any browned bits from the bottom of the pan. Simmer until the liquid is slightly thickened, 5 to 10 minutes. Cut the chicken into quarters and serve each with the pan sauce and a cherry pepper.

MAKES 2 SERVINGS, WITH LEFTOVERS · PER SERVING **369** CALORIES // **17 G** FAT // **970 MG** SODIUM // **3 G** CARBOHYDRATES // **1 G** DIETARY FIBER // **48 G** PROTEIN

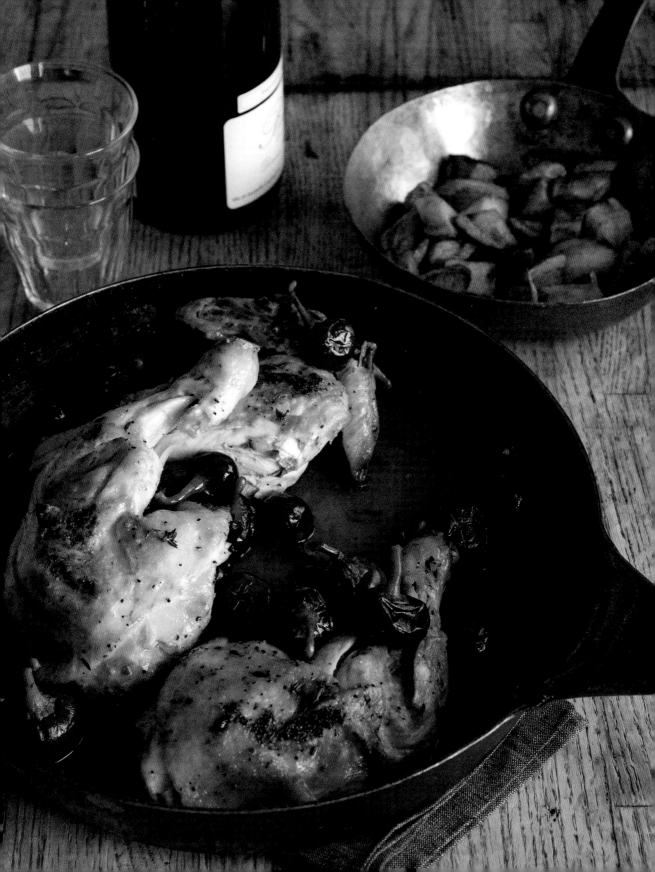

CHOCOLATE POT DE CRÈME

This sensual dessert mimics chocolate mousse, but is far simpler to prepare. Serve it to her with a glass of champagne after a night out (it needs to chill in the fridge for a few hours anyway). The best part? There aren't even 200 calories in one serving. So go ahead and sample a couple before she comes over.

1	tablespoon sugar
1	tablespoon unsweetened cocoa powder
	Pinch of salt
3	ounces bittersweet chocolate, chopped into small pieces (do not use unsweetened chocolate)
⅓	cup half-and-half
2	tablespoons brewed espresso
¼	teaspoon vanilla extract
1	egg, whisked
¼	cup whipped cream

1. In a medium microwaveable bowl, stir together the sugar, cocoa powder, and salt. Add the chocolate, half-and-half, espresso, and vanilla extract. Microwave on high for 1 minute. Whisk, microwave for 30 seconds longer, and whisk again. The chocolate should be completely melted, and the liquid should be very hot but not boiling. Pour into a blender. Blend, slowly adding the egg, for about 1 minute.

2. Pour about ⅓ cup into each of 4 ramekins, bowls, or small teacups. Refrigerate for at least 4 hours.

3. Top each serving with 1 tablespoon whipped cream.

MAKES 4 SERVINGS · PER SERVING 171 CALORIES // 14 G FAT // 38 MG SODIUM // 16 G CARBOHYDRATES // 2 G DIETARY FIBER // 3 G PROTEIN

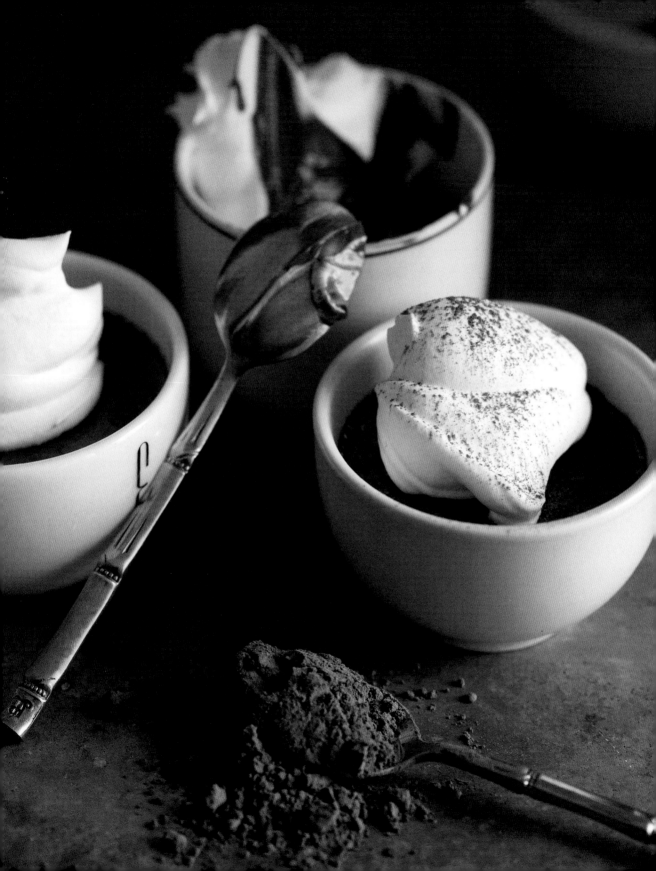

LEMON SEMIFREDDO
with STRAWBERRIES

Dessert is where an otherwise exemplary meal can jump off the rails.
This refreshing semifreddo requires minimal prep, but tastes like
you've been slaving away in the kitchen all day just for her.

---

1   pint strawberries, thinly sliced

2   tablespoons sugar

½   cup heavy cream

½   cup store-bought lemon curd

     Shortbread cookies (optional)

1. Place the strawberries in a bowl. Add the sugar and toss once or twice. Cover the bowl with plastic wrap and let the berries sit at room temperature until they release their juices, at least 30 minutes. (You can do this several hours ahead and refrigerate the fruit until ready to use.)

2. In a large metal mixing bowl, whisk the heavy cream until thickened. (Use an electric mixer if you own one, or the biggest whisk you can find.) Add the lemon curd and stir until just combined. Divide the mixture between two small bowls, cover with plastic, and chill in the freezer until thickened to an ice cream consistency, at least 1 hour.

3. To serve, spoon some berries over the semifreddo and then garnish with shortbread cookies, if you like.

MAKES 2 SERVINGS · PER SERVING **522** CALORIES // **2 G** FAT // **94 MG** SODIUM // **79 G** CARBOHYDRATES // **3 G** DIETARY FIBER // **2 G** PROTEIN

ICE CREAM AFFOGATO

This recipe's genius comes from combining hot and cold, sweet and bitter, all by using just three ingredients. Think quality here. Seek out the best espresso you can find and buy a high-grade vanilla ice cream (the fewer ingredients on the label, the better). The extra cash you drop will far outweigh the fact that this dessert takes almost no time to assemble.

1	cup vanilla ice cream
1	tablespoon Kahlúa coffee liqueur
4	tablespoons hot espresso

Divide the ice cream between two small dessert bowls. Stir the liqueur into the espresso, and then pour over the ice cream. Serve immediately.

MAKES 2 SERVINGS · PER SERVING **166** CALORIES // **7 G** FAT // **58 MG** SODIUM // **19 G** CARBOHYDRATES // **0 G** DIETARY FIBER // **2 G** PROTEIN

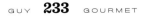

ICE CREAM SAUCES

What woman doesn't love ice cream?
Do this: Buy a great vanilla ice cream, then simmer
a sweet sauce to drizzle over the scoops.

FRESH STRAWBERRY SAUCE

1   cup chopped
     strawberries

2 to 3 tablespoons sugar,
     to taste

½   teaspoon orange liqueur

In a medium bowl, combine all
of the ingredients and mash the
strawberries until the sauce is
mostly smooth. Let stand about
10 minutes before serving.

MAPLE-WALNUT SAUCE

¼   cup maple syrup

1   tablespoon rum

2   tablespoons chopped
     toasted walnuts

In a small saucepan, combine
the maple syrup and rum and
simmer until reduced by half.
Stir in the walnuts and serve
warm.

CHOCOLATE-COFFEE SAUCE

3   ounces semisweet
     chocolate, coarsely
     chopped

1   tablespoon black coffee

¼   cup heavy cream

1½   teaspoons butter

In a microwaveable bowl,
combine the chocolate, coffee,
and cream. Microwave until
the chocolate is mostly
melted—1 to 2 minutes—
stirring halfway through. Stir
in the butter until smooth.

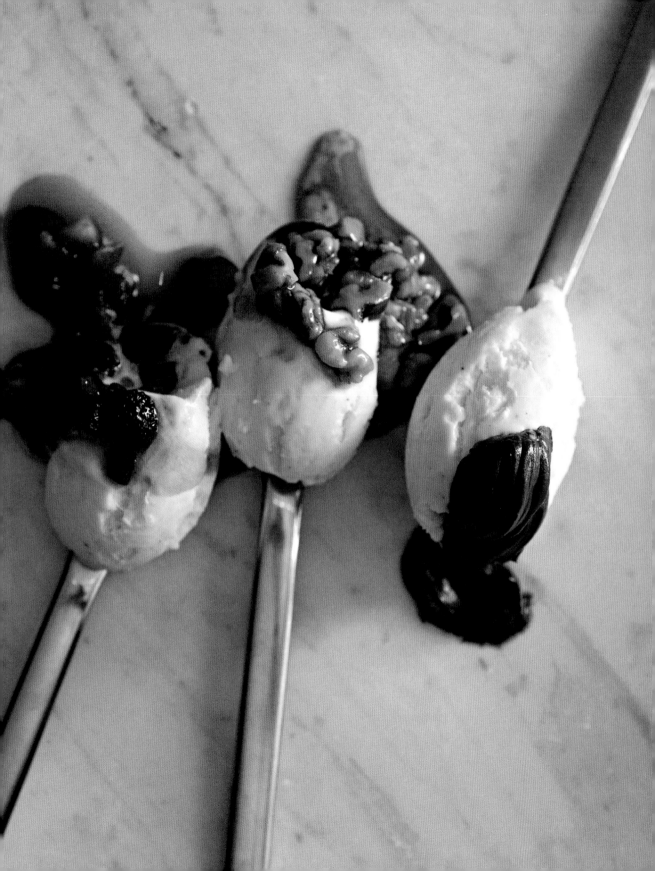

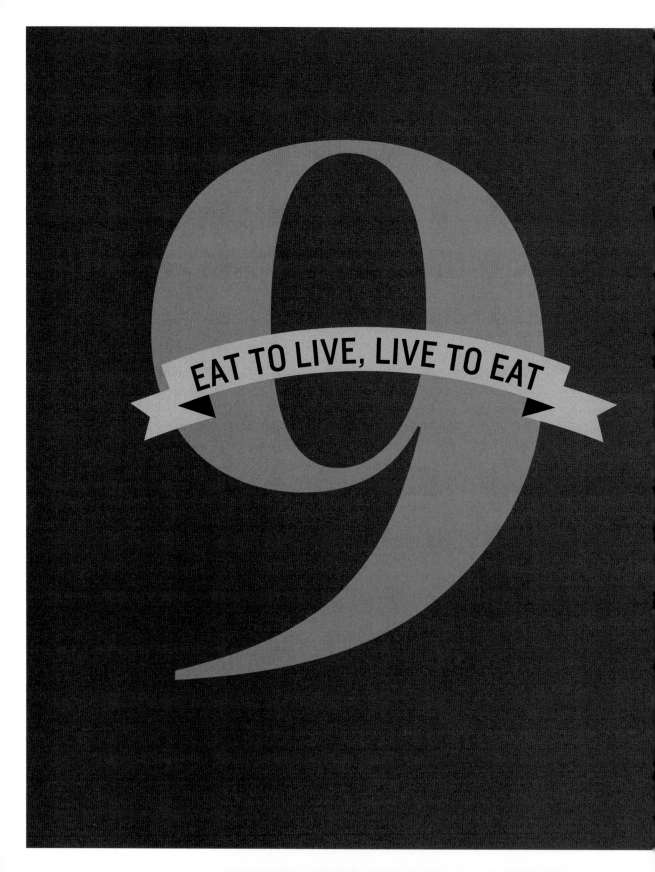

9

EAT TO LIVE, LIVE TO EAT

CELEBRATION
MEALS

Party smarter with holiday meals that won't wipe you out or weigh you down.

p. 238   GUY MH GOURMET   c. 09

THE RULES *of* HOLIDAY COOKING

When you cook for a celebration, you have an audience waiting to be impressed. So don't dump soup mix into sour cream and call it a day. Pull off an element of a big feast, and folks will be dishing up compliments long after dessert.

RULE N⁰.

1

TAKE COMMAND OF YOUR KITCHEN

IF YOU CAN help out with the menu at a holiday celebration, you decide what goes into your stomach. That goes for feeding your family or friends at your place, but also bringing along a dish to someone else's party. We've packed this chapter with main courses, side dishes, and, yes, even desserts, that taste like indulgences and won't end up busting your gut. So while you may be walking into a holiday bacchanal loaded with empty-calorie dishes, at least you'll be carrying a go-to that has gut-filling fibrous vegetables and/ or lean protein.

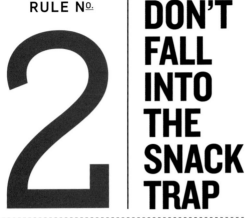

2

DON'T FALL INTO THE SNACK TRAP

THE HORS D'OEUVRES table is that seemingly innocent siren of the holiday party. Cheese, crackers, dips, those mini hot dogs wrapped in pastry dough—how harmful could it be to just have a few bites, right? Then, before you know it, you're searching for the nearest couch, bogged down by calories, and wondering if you can pull off a party nap. To avoid the bloat (and the embarrassment), choose the one law of the hors d'oeuvre spread: Pick only the foods that contain high amounts of fiber (that veggie tray, those prosciutto-wrapped asparagus spears) or pure protein (shrimp skewers, bacon-wrapped scallops). Have one or two of each, and then back away from the buffet table. These foods contain gut-filling abilities that can actually help you consume fewer calories when dinner finally rolls around. Just don't overdo it.

3

WATCH THE DRINKABLE CALORIES

YOU KNOW THAT Aunt Erma calls it "sinful" triple chocolate cake for a reason, so you can avoid it easier. But sneakier calories can catch you off guard if you're not careful—namely those hiding out in the beer bucket. Check out this list of the caloric values of common brews to prevent a caloric beer bomb.

LEANEST	CALORIES	CARBS (G)
BUDWEISER SELECT	55	2
MILLER LIGHT	96	3
MOLSON CANADIAN LIGHT	113	10
MOLSON CANADIAN	136	11
PABST BLUE RIBBON	144	13
BUDWEISER	145	11
GUINNESS EXTRA STOUT	176	14
BLUE MOON BELGIAN WHITE	184	13
HURRICANE HIGH GRAVITY	188	7
SIERRA NEVADA BIGFOOT	330	32
MEANEST		

BONUS TIP: To help stave off chain-drinking, fend off a hangover, and keep yourself hydrated, always chase a serving of alcohol with 8 ounces of water. You'll thank us in the morning.

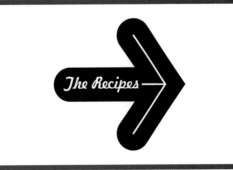

The Recipes →

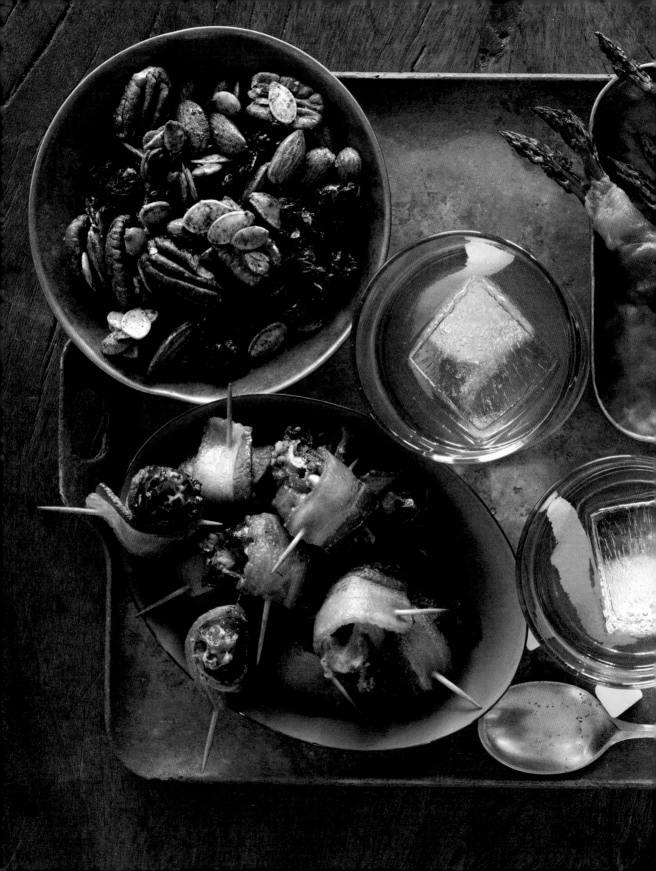

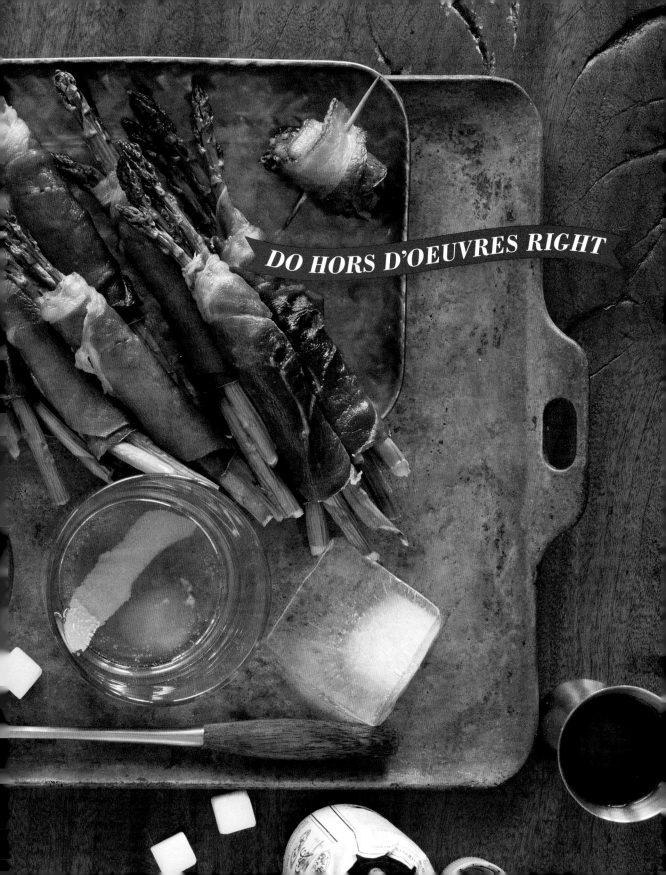

DO HORS D'OEUVRES RIGHT

DATES WITH BACON

These delicacies from Seamus Mullen, chef and partner at New York tapas hot spot Boqueria, are perfect for handing off to your guests. They're sweet, savory, and nutty—all rolled, literally, into one awesome appetizer.

---

18 large Medjool dates, pitted

18 Marcona almonds

¼ pound Valdeón cheese (or another mild blue cheese)

9 slices bacon, each slice cut in half crosswise

Preheat the oven to 425°F. Stuff each date with a Marcona almond and ½ tablespoon Valdeón cheese. Wrap with a piece of bacon and skewer with a toothpick. Bake on a baking sheet until the bacon is golden brown, 5 to 7 minutes.

MAKES 18 SERVINGS · PER SERVING **124** CALORIES // **5 G** FAT // **141 MG** SODIUM // **18 G** CARBOHYDRATES // **2 G** DIETARY FIBER // **3 G** PROTEIN

PROSCIUTTO-WRAPPED ASPARAGUS WITH DIJON

Tender, vibrant asparagus melds with salty mustard and cured pork in a meal-starter that your guests are likely to chow down on faster than it took you to cook up.

1   **bunch thin asparagus, ends trimmed**

     Olive oil

     Freshly ground black pepper

4   **ounces thin-sliced prosciutto, slices cut into thirds lengthwise**

1. Preheat the oven to 375°F. Place the asparagus on a large baking sheet. Drizzle with olive oil and season with pepper. Mix with your hands until the asparagus is evenly covered.

2. Wrap 1 slice of prosciutto around 2 or 3 asparagus stalks. Return the bundle to the baking sheet. Repeat, evenly spacing the asparagus on the pan.

3. Bake until the prosciutto starts crisping and the asparagus is crisp-tender, about 15 minutes. Cut each asparagus bundle in half on the bias before serving.

MAKES 4 SERVINGS · PER 5-SPEAR SERVING **97** CALORIES // **5 G** FAT // **761 MG** SODIUM // **4 G** CARBOHYDRATES // **2 G** DIETARY FIBER // **10 G** PROTEIN

HORS D'OEUVRES

SPICY COCKTAIL NUTS

Not only to pair with beer at parties, these spicy nuts can be stashed in resealable plastic bags for snacking at work.

1	cup hulled pumpkin seeds
1	teaspoon canola oil
1	cup almonds
1	cup pecan halves
2	tablespoons maple syrup
½	teaspoon ground allspice
½	teaspoon ground cinnamon
½	teaspoon ground nutmeg
½	teaspoon sea salt
1	cup orange-flavored dried cranberries

1. Preheat the oven to 350°F. Coat a rimmed baking sheet with nonstick spray. In a bowl, toss the pumpkin seeds with the oil to coat. Spread the seeds on the baking sheet and bake for about 20 minutes, stirring several times. Remove the pumpkin seeds but leave the oven on.

2. Place the pumpkin seeds, almonds, and pecans in a medium bowl and stir in the maple syrup to coat. In a small bowl, mix together the allspice, cinnamon, nutmeg, and salt. Add to the nuts and stir well.

3. Spread the mixture on the baking sheet and bake, stirring occasionally, until dry, about 15 minutes. Check often to avoid burning. Cool in the pan for 20 minutes.

4. Transfer the cooled mix to a bowl and stir in the cranberries.

MAKES 12 SERVINGS · PER SERVING **256** CALORIES // **20 G** FAT // **99 MG** SODIUM // **16 G** CARBOHYDRATES // **3 G** DIETARY FIBER // **7 G** PROTEIN

BABY-SPINACH SALAD *with* GOAT CHEESE *and* PISTACHIOS

Holiday meals should start off simple, yet impressive enough to set the tone of the meal to come. Serve guests this palate-primer that matches the lightness of baby spinach with the creaminess of goat cheese.

½ cup balsamic vinegar

¼ cup extra-virgin olive oil

Dash of salt

Dash of ground black pepper

16 cups loosely packed baby spinach

½ pound goat cheese, crumbled

½ cup pistachios, toasted

1. In a large bowl, whisk together the vinegar and oil. Season with the salt and pepper.

2. Add the spinach to the vinaigrette and toss, using tongs to coat the spinach evenly. Divide the spinach among plates and top with the cheese and nuts.

MAKES 8 SERVINGS · PER SERVING 231 CALORIES // 18 G FAT // 305 MG SODIUM // 10 G CARBOHYDRATES // 3 G DIETARY FIBER // 9 G PROTEIN

o PARMESAN CRISPS

Grate enough Parmesan to completely cover a small, round, microwaveable plate. Microwave on high until the cheese is crisp, about 80 seconds. Remove the plate and let it sit for about 10 seconds; then peel the cheese from the plate and serve it with Caesar salad or as a garnish for soups.

SQUASH-APPLE SOUP

Skip the heavy creamed soups and whip up this produce-based alternative. It's still creamy, but that's because of the squash puree. You'll leave your guests ready for the next course, not already stuffed.

1	**tablespoon vegetable oil**
2	**shallots, chopped**
1	**tablespoon minced fresh ginger**
2	**packages (12 ounces each) frozen squash puree, thawed**
3	**cups reduced-sodium vegetable broth**
1	**apple, diced**
1	**tablespoon dried sage**
	Salt and ground black pepper
	Sour cream, for serving

Heat the oil in a large saucepan over medium heat. Add the shallots and ginger and cook for 3 minutes. Add the squash puree, vegetable broth, apple, sage, and salt and pepper to taste. Bring to a boil, then simmer, covered, for 15 minutes. In batches, process the soup in a blender until smooth. Serve with a swirl of sour cream.

MAKES 4 SERVINGS · PER SERVING **171** CALORIES // **3.5 G** FAT // **145 MG** SODIUM // **37 G** CARBOHYDRATES // **4 G** DIETARY FIBER // **4 G** PROTEIN

GUINNESS-BRAISED SHORT RIBS

Beer and beef make a masterful match in this easy, hearty, slow-cooker stew. Stuff all the ingredients into a slow cooker in the afternoon; pull them out when your friends or family arrive. Holiday stress? What holiday stress?

2	pounds boneless beef short ribs
	Salt and ground black pepper
1	tablespoon canola oil
2	cans or bottles Guinness Draught
2	cups beef broth
3	large carrots, cut into large chunks
2	onions, quartered
2	ribs celery, cut into large chunks
8	cloves garlic, peeled
2	bay leaves

1. Season the short ribs with salt and pepper to taste. Heat the oil in a large sauté pan over high heat. When the oil is hot, add the ribs and cook them, turning occasionally, until they're browned all over, about 10 minutes. Transfer the ribs to a slow cooker.

2. While the pan is still hot, deglaze it by pouring in the beer and scraping up any browned bits. Then pour the beer and bits over the ribs in the slow cooker.

3. Add the remaining ingredients to the slow cooker and turn it on high. Cook the ribs until they're nearly falling apart, about 4 hours. Serve the stew over soft polenta or mashed potatoes.

MAKES 4 SERVINGS · PER SERVING 574 CALORIES // 27 G FAT // 684 MG SODIUM // 22 G CARBOHYDRATES // 3.5 G DIETARY FIBER // 48 G PROTEIN

PEAR-STUFFED PORK ROAST

A large piece of meat feeds a crowd with ease, but you need to infuse flavor from the inside out. The fix: Use a basic butcher technique to fill the tenderloin with a fruit-based stuffing. This recipe comes from Adam Sappington, chef at The Country Cat in Portland.

1	boneless center-cut pork loin roast (4 pounds)
2	tablespoons thyme salt (equal amounts of dried thyme and kosher salt)
3	tablespoons unsalted butter
⅓	pound ham, coarsely chopped
3	shallots, thinly sliced
2	Bosc pears, peeled and diced
1	cup apple cider
	Leaves from 1 bunch of fresh thyme, chopped
3	sprigs fresh rosemary
3	fennel fronds
3	onions, cut into quarters, with onion layers separated

1. Thoroughly massage the pork with the thyme salt. Place it on a baking rack and refrigerate it overnight.

2. An hour before cooking the pork, take it out of the fridge. Preheat the oven to 375°F. Melt the butter in a large sauté pan over medium heat. Add the ham and cook until caramelized, 15 to 20 minutes. Add the shallots and cook until golden, 5 minutes. Add the pears and cook until softened, 15 minutes. Add the cider, increase the heat to high, and cook until the stuffing is chunky. Chill it on a baking sheet for 15 minutes.

3. Stuff the pork loin (see "How to Stuff a Tenderloin," below). On a foil-lined rimmed baking sheet, place the fresh thyme, rosemary, fennel, and onions and top with the pork. Roast until an instant-read thermometer inserted in the center reads 140°F. Transfer the pork to a cutting board and let it rest for 5 minutes before slicing.

MAKES 8 SERVINGS · PER SERVING **379** CALORIES // **10 G** FAT // **730 MG** SODIUM // **19 G** CARBOHYDRATES // **2 G** DIETARY FIBER // **52 G** PROTEIN

○ HOW TO STUFF A TENDERLOIN

1. Insert a long, thin slicing knife into the middle of one end of the roast as far as you can. Repeat on the other end to form a tunnel. Move the knife back and forth to enlarge the hole.

2. Transfer the chilled stuffing to a resealable plastic bag and cut off one of the corners to create a 1½" hole, making a jury-rigged piping bag. Insert the "tip" of the piping bag into one end of the loin, grip the open end of the bag, and squeeze the filling into the loin. Turn the loin and stuff it from the other end.

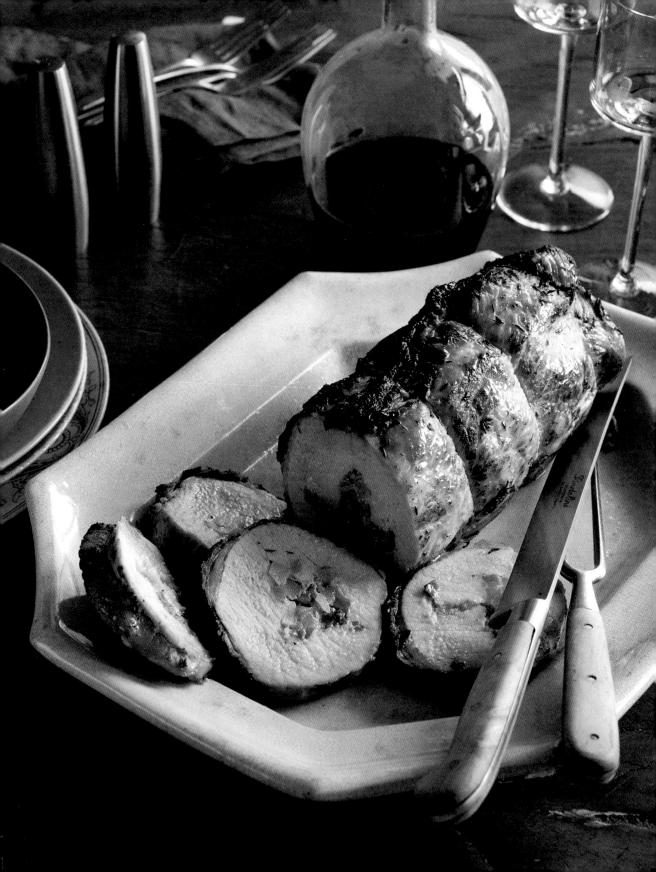

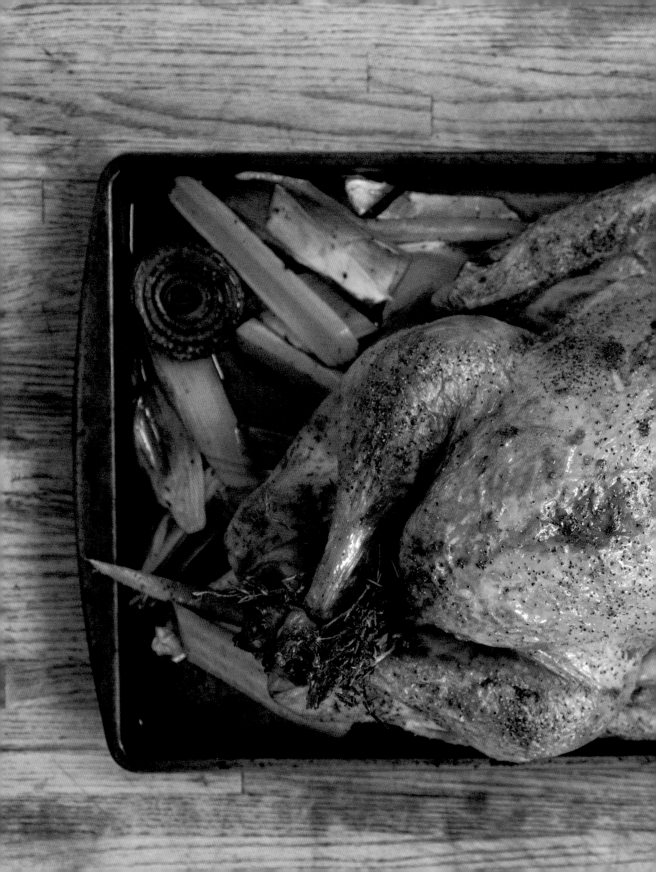

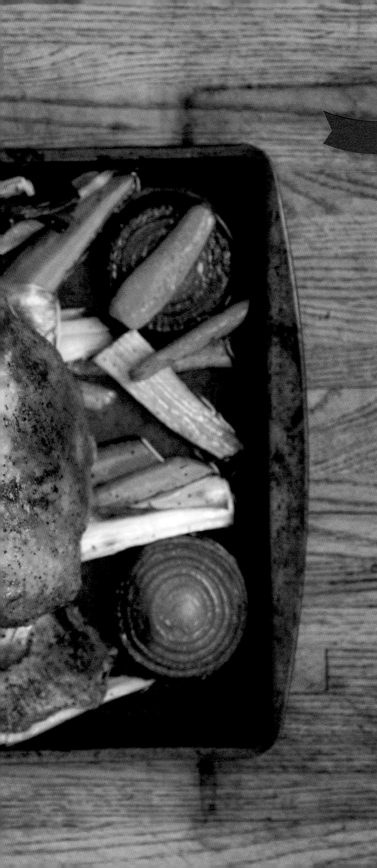

THANKSGIVING

CLASSIC TURKEY

and

STUFFING

DON'T BRINE IT, SALT IT!

Salting your bird ahead of time adds flavor and moisture, but there's no need to bother with sloppy brining—just salt the turkey a couple of days before cooking. Remove the giblets and rub the bird inside and out with kosher salt—about 1 tablespoon per 5 pounds of bird. You can mix a rounded teaspoon of ancho chile powder into the salt to give the bird a little smoky sweetness. Chill the turkey, wrapped in a plastic turkey bag, until the big day.

DON'T STUFF IT

Yes, stuffing is delicious, but because it inhibits air circulation, it slows cooking, and to heat it sufficiently to serve it safely, you might need to cook the bird more than is advantageous. If you really want to put something in the cavity, throw a handful of herbs and a halved onion in there. You can cook stuffing separately, dousing it with more stock and butter than if you were roasting it in the bird. See "The Easiest Turkey Day Stuffing" for a simple recipe.

WHO NEEDS A RACK?

If you're only an occasional meat roaster, you can skip the roasting pan and rack. Equip yourself instead with a cheap but sturdy sheet pan, and give your bird some air circulation with a foundation of chunked-up vegetables, all cut in 2" to 4" pieces. Put down a layer of a couple of peeled carrots, a couple of onions, a rib of celery, and a leek if you have it. Put the turkey, breast side up, on top of the veggies. As it roasts, they will also give the pan drippings extra flavor.

BASTE NOT

Basting's a nice way to feel like you're tending to your turkey, but it is an easy way to burn yourself, and it causes the oven to lose a lot of heat. In the end it doesn't make a huge difference in the bird—so feel free to skip it. You'd rather be tossing the football, right?

BUY A NEW THERMOMETER

And use it. Just because your bird is golden-brown doesn't mean it's not raw inside. And for even cooking, start by removing the turkey from the fridge 1 hour before it hits the oven. Preheat the oven to 425°F. Pat the turkey dry with paper towels and give it a quick massage with a tablespoon or two of olive oil. Then put it in a roasting pan filled with vegetables and roast for 30 minutes. Turn down the oven to 325°F and continue roasting until a thermometer inserted at the thickest part of the turkey thigh reads 165°F. Let the bird rest at least 30 to 50 minutes before carving. While it's resting, bake the stuffing.

LAYAWAY GRAVY

Make your gravy ahead of time and avoid the potential stress of last-minute gravy whisking. In a saucepan, combine 1 cup of white wine, 1 minced onion, and a few sprigs of tarragon and boil together until the wine has completely evaporated. Discard the tarragon, scoop the onions out of the pan and save them, and then melt 4 tablespoons of butter with 4 tablespoons of flour over medium-low heat. Cook for a few minutes without browning, and then pour in 3 cups warm chicken stock. Whisk thoroughly and turn up the heat to bring to a boil, then turn down the heat and cook for a couple of minutes until the sauce thickens, then add the onions. Cook gently for another 5 minutes and season with salt and a touch of black pepper.

Refrigerate the gravy until Thanksgiving, when you can reheat it. To add extra flavor, remove the veggies from the hot turkey pan and deglaze it with a splash of wine, scraping up any browned bits with a wooden spoon. Stir into the gravy. Strain if you prefer a smooth sauce, or serve it a little chunky.

THE EASIEST TURKEY DAY STUFFING

1	tablespoon olive oil
2	large onions, chopped
2	large ribs celery, chopped
2	teaspoons poultry seasoning
3	cups turkey or chicken stock
1	pound day-old sourdough bread, cut into cubes
¾	cup chopped fresh parsley
4	tablespoons (½ stick) unsalted butter, melted
	Salt and ground black pepper

Preheat the oven to 350°F. Heat the oil in large pot over medium heat. Add the onions, celery, and poultry seasoning. Cook until softened, about 6 minutes. Add the turkey stock and bring to a simmer. Remove the pan from the heat and stir in the bread, parsley, and butter, tossing to combine well. Season the stuffing and transfer to an oiled 3-quart baking dish. Cover with foil and bake for 20 minutes; uncover and continue to bake until nicely browned, about 20 minutes more.

MAKES 12 SERVINGS · PER SERVING 172 CALORIES // 5 G FAT // 375 MG SODIUM // 25 G CARBOHYDRATES // 2 G DIETARY FIBER // 6 G PROTEIN

THANKSGIVING

THE BEST WAY TO CARVE A TURKEY?

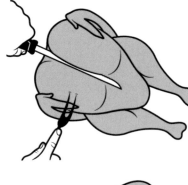

DON'T CARVE AT THE TABLE

"To do it right, you need to manhandle the carcass," says Alton Brown, the host of Food Network's *Good Eats*. "That means working in the kitchen, where you can get hands-on without an audience."

BE PATIENT

Your best defense against dry meat is to let the turkey sit for at least 30 minutes before carving. This allows the flesh to reabsorb juices. "Plus, who can carve a rocket-hot turkey?" says Brown.

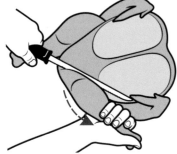

THINK BIG

The aim is to remove each breast in one solid piece, says Brown. Cut down on either side of the keelbone—the big bone that sticks up between the breasts—until you hit where the rib cage turns out. Then turn the knife outward and keep cutting until you have a teardrop-shaped slab. Set it aside and carve off the other breast.

FLIP THE BIRD

Turn the turkey over so its underside faces up. "Grab the thigh and bend it backward to pop the socket," Brown says. When you hear it snap, use the knife to separate the thigh from the rest of the bird. Next, cut the drumstick away from the thigh. The drumsticks can be served as they are. Use the same bend-and-cut technique on the wings.

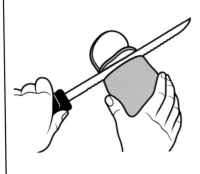

SLICE AWAY

To cut the thigh, hold it upright (perpendicular to the board) and slice downward, moving around the bone. Then place the breast on the cutting board skin side up. Cut it like you would a loaf of bread, into slices about ⅓" thick. "This way you're cutting against the grain, which runs the length of the breast, and it's going to be more tender, because the meat fibers are shorter," says Brown.

TURKEY IN A TRASH CAN

Roast turkey takes forever and monopolizes valuable oven space. Fried turkey is, well, fried. But trash-can turkey frees up Thanksgiving kitchen real estate, cooks quickly, and tastes incredible. Seriously.

1 turkey (about a 12-pounder), thawed, giblets packet removed, and rinsed

Olive oil

¼ cup chopped fresh rosemary

Salt and ground black pepper

EQUIPMENT

New steel trash can (20-gallon size)

Aluminum foil (two rolls of extra-wide)

Charcoal briquettes (three 10-pound bags)

Newspaper

Lighter fluid

Matches

Hammer

Broom handle or sturdy stick (2 feet long)

Large metal shovel

Heatproof gloves

Meat thermometer

Bucket of water

Fire extinguisher

PREP THE TURKEY

Rub the turkey with olive oil and rosemary; season all over with salt and pepper.

SECURE YOUR SITE

Clear a fire pit of any rocks, twigs, or other debris, and line it with foil.

CLEAN THE CAN

Using a clean scrub brush and hot soapy water, thoroughly clean and rinse the inside of the can.

LIGHT THE COALS

Mold a few sheets of foil so they form a bowl large enough to hold about 1½ bags of charcoal. Place the bowl in the fire pit, off to the side. Line the bowl with several sheets of newspaper, fill it with charcoal, add lighter fluid, and light the paper. The coals are ready when they're covered with ash, after about 20 minutes.

MAKE THE OVEN

While the coals are heating, hammer the broom handle securely into the dirt in the center of the fire pit. Then shove a wad of foil into the turkey's cavity and balance the bird on the stick. Gently place the can over the bird.

TURN ON THE HEAT

Shovel a ring of coals against the trash can's base, and the remaining coals on top of the can. Let the turkey cook until the charcoal turns to ash, about 2 hours. If the coals turn to ash and start to cool before 2 hours, shovel on a fresh layer of coals. The heat from the smoldering briquettes will light the new ones.

Important: Do not lift the can to check on the turkey. Valuable heat will escape from the trash can, and the turkey will require much more time to cook.

REMOVE AND EAT

Using heatproof gloves, lift the hot can off the cooked bird. Stick the turkey with a meat thermometer—if it reads 165°F at the thigh, it's safe to eat. Douse the coals with water, being cautious of the resulting smoke or ash.

CHILI-SPICED MASHED SWEET POTATOES

You don't need those little marshmallows. Instead, deploy fresh orange juice, a little orange zest, and some chili powder to give it zing.

4	large sweet potatoes (3½ pounds total)
2	teaspoons grated orange zest
½	cup fresh orange juice
2	tablespoons light brown sugar
2	teaspoons ground cinnamon
1	teaspoon chili powder
¼	teaspoon salt

1. Preheat the oven to 425°F. Bake the sweet potatoes until they are soft, about 1 hour 10 minutes. Remove from the oven and let cool slightly.

2. In a small bowl, whisk together the orange zest, orange juice, brown sugar, cinnamon, chili powder, and salt.

3. Scoop the sweet potato flesh into a large bowl. Pour in the orange juice mixture and mash well.

MAKES 8 SERVINGS · PER SERVING **194** CALORIES // **0 G** FAT // **186 MG** SODIUM // **46 G** CARBOHYDRATES // **6 G** DIETARY FIBER // **3 G** PROTEIN

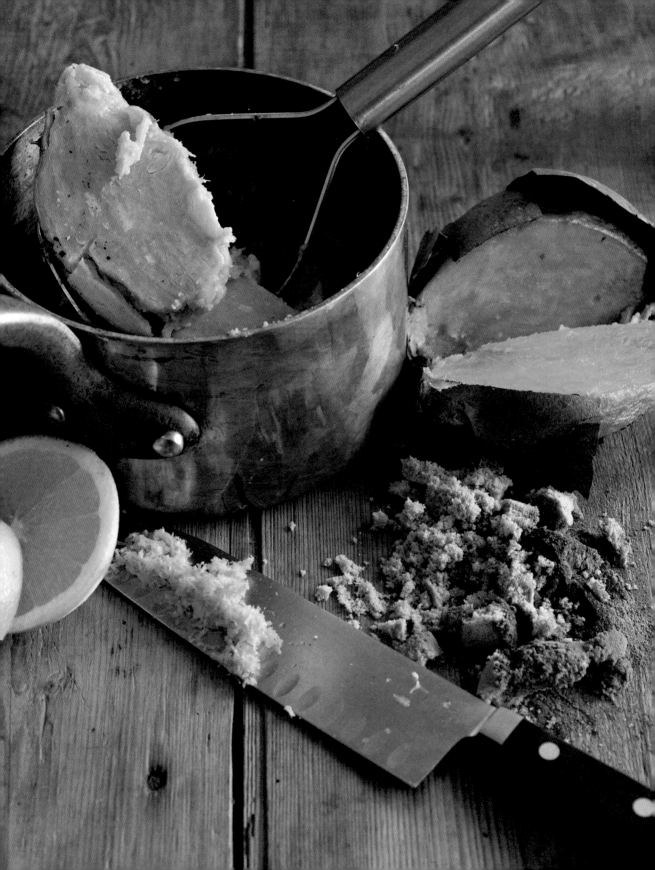

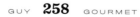

HEALTHIER GREEN BEAN CASSEROLE

It's a new twist on that old-fashioned favorite from Thanksgivings past. Next time you're headed to a holiday potluck, bring this dish and you'll have a simple, impressive dish that'll have the other guests begging for the recipe.

½ cup buttermilk

½ cup plain dry bread crumbs

1 onion, cut crosswise into ¼"-thick slices and separated into rings

8 ounces mushrooms, sliced

1 small onion, chopped

½ teaspoon dried thyme

¼ teaspoon salt

¼ cup unbleached or all-purpose flour

3 cups 1% milk

1 bag (16 ounces) frozen French-cut green beans, thawed and drained

1. Preheat the oven to 500°F. Coat a medium baking dish with nonstick spray. Coat a baking sheet with nonstick spray.

2. Place the buttermilk in a shallow bowl. Place the bread crumbs in another shallow bowl. Dip the onion rings into the buttermilk, then dredge in the bread crumbs and place on the baking sheet. Coat lightly with nonstick spray. Bake until tender and golden brown, about 20 minutes. Remove from the oven and leave the oven on, but reduce the temperature to 400°F.

3. Meanwhile, coat a medium saucepan with nonstick spray. Set over medium heat. Add the mushrooms, chopped onion, thyme, and salt. Coat with nonstick spray. Cook, stirring occasionally, for 4 to 5 minutes, or until the mushrooms give off liquid. Sprinkle with the flour. Cook, stirring, for 1 minute. Add the milk. Cook, stirring constantly, until thickened, 3 to 4 minutes. Add the green beans. Stir to mix.

4. Pour the bean mixture into the prepared baking dish. Scatter the onion rings over the top. Bake until hot and bubbling, 25 to 30 minutes.

MAKES 6 SERVINGS · PER SERVING 121 CALORIES // **2 G** FAT // **184 MG** SODIUM // **21 G** CARBOHYDRATES // **3 G** DIETARY FIBER // **7 G** PROTEIN

BAKED APPLES

Don't load down your holiday dinners with icing-laden cakes and trays of cookies. Instead, opt for this simple bake-and-serve dessert that won't leave your guests in a postmeal couch coma.

4	Rome or Gala apples
	Grated zest and juice of 1 lemon
½	cup raisins, coarsely chopped
¼	cup chopped toasted walnuts
¼	cup packed light brown sugar
1	tablespoon Cognac (optional)
1	teaspoon ground cinnamon
¼	teaspoon ground cloves
1½	teaspoons cornstarch
1½	cups orange juice

1. Preheat the oven to 350°F.

2. Using a corer or paring knife, make a 1"-diameter hole through the core of each apple. Place the apples, right side up, in a 9" x 9" baking dish.

3. In a medium bowl, combine the lemon zest, lemon juice, raisins, walnuts, brown sugar, Cognac (if using), cinnamon, and cloves. Spoon into the apples.

4. Place the cornstarch in a small bowl. Add the orange juice and stir until smooth. Pour around the apples.

5. Bake, occasionally basting the apples with the pan juices, until softened, 50 to 60 minutes. Serve warm.

MAKES 4 SERVINGS · PER SERVING 206 CALORIES // 5 G FAT // 10 MG SODIUM // 68 G CARBOHYDRATES // 6 G DIETARY FIBER // 3 G PROTEIN

CREATE A CHEESE PLATTER

Look beyond the singles and strings and into the gourmet cheese section of your supermarket (or check out artisanalcheese.com), and use our guide to discover the best cheeses you aren't eating.

ROBIOLA
SUPERSPREAD

Step away from the Cheez Whiz: Robiola is the best way to top a Triscuit. This Italian cheese is soft, like Brie, and it tastes as rich as butter. Spread it on a whole grain cracker or baguette slice, and round out the snack with grapes or cantaloupe. For another great spread, try Brillat-Savarin, which is so creamy it's been called the cheese equivalent of ice cream.

RONCAL
ANYTIME SNACK

A firm sheep's-milk cheese, Roncal's nutty flavor and chewy texture make it a fine stand-alone snack. Or, to add a touch of sweetness, you can give it a light glaze of cherry or raspberry preserves. A delicious alternative is Comté, one of the most popular cheeses in France. Besides being a great snack, Comté can also be a tasty filling for a grilled-cheese sandwich.

SAINTE-MAURE
SALAD ENHANCER

This French goat cheese makes any salad taste better. But don't try to crumble Sainte-Maure like you would other kinds of goat cheese—it's too soft. Instead, serve it on the side of a mixed-greens salad. For the dressing, combine 2 tablespoons sherry vinegar, ⅓ cup walnut oil, 1 tablespoon finely diced shallots, 1 teaspoon kosher salt, and some black pepper. Nab a bit of cheese with your fork, stab some lettuce, and bite down. The lemon and black pepper flavors of the cheese blend perfectly with the earthy walnut oil.

AGED GOUDA
FLAVOR KING

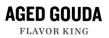

Most cheeses can be aged for weeks to months, but a well-produced Gouda has spent 3 to 5 years in a cave. "Cheese is aged to develop its flavors," says Scott A. Rankin, Ph.D., an associate professor of food science at the University of Wisconsin at Madison. The result is like a good Parmigiano Reggiano, but with rich caramel flavors. Eat thin slices with a green apple or pear.

MONTGOMERY'S CHEDDAR
BEER BUDDY

Don't expect this cheese to taste like the factory-formed orange bricks you find in your supermarket. This is authentic cheddar, from Manor Farm in Somerset, the county in England where the cheese originated. Its lingering flavors of buttermilk and horseradish balance well with any beer and make American cheddar seem bland.

HOJA SANTA
WINE COMPANION

This creamy goat cheese from Texas is wrapped in leaves of hoja santa, an herb that imparts licorice and mint flavors. Serve it with a sauvignon blanc. White wine is usually a better complement to a cheese plate than red is, because its acidity balances the fat. Another one to eat with vino is Cypress Grove Chevre Purple Haze, a goat cheese from northern California.

BAYLEY HAZEN BLUE
DESSERT CHEESE

This Vermont blue cheese tastes like chocolate. The fudgelike flavor even has a hint of apricot. Eat it alone, or drizzle a drop or two of honey on it for an even sweeter (but still healthy) treat.

THE BEST MAIL-ORDER MEATS

We searched for the nation's best mail-order meats. Just wait for the big brown van, and then feed your muscles some top-quality protein.

1 BLOC DE FOIE GRAS DE CANARD

This duck-liver delicacy is smooth like velvet, with hints of Cognac and spices. Spread it on whole wheat crackers—from 3pigs.com.

2 SURRYANO HAM

It comes from a rare breed of hog. Eat it as is, or wrap slices, like prosciutto, around melon wedges—from surryfarms.com.

3 FENNEL SALAMI

The fennel flavor melds with either brown sugar or orange zest during a slow-curing process that requires less salt—from boccalone.com.

4 NDUJA

For an appetizer, try this spicy, spreadable salami on toasted baguette rounds—from boccalone.com.

5 SNAKE RIVER FARMS AMERICAN WAGYU BEEF

From a hybrid of Japanese Kobe cattle: same tenderness, but one-quarter the price—from snakeriverfarms.com.

6 JAMISON FARM LAMB

Many top restaurant chefs serve this same lamb. Rub it with spices and salt before cooking—from jamisonfarm.com.

7 LIBERTY DUCKS BREAST FILLETS

Before roasting, score them and melt off some of the fat by searing in oil, skin side down, for 10 minutes—from libertyducks.com.

NUTRITION

BE MERRY WITHOUT THE BELLY

Tips that will get you through holiday parties without moving up a pants size

'Tis the season for spending time with friends, coworkers, neighbors, and family—and, of course, "spending time" translates into eating food. A lot of it. But don't resign yourself to a winter of baggy sweatshirts or wait until January to worry about your newly acquired gut. The No. 1 mistake people make during the holidays is self-sabotage, according to Jim White, spokesman for the American Dietetic Association. "[Gyms nationwide] are slammed the whole month of January," White says. "If you can lose weight by January 1, you'll beat the crowds." Not to mention look good in all those pictures.

1

BUDGET YOUR CALORIES

If you're heading to a party and know you'll be surrounded by food, prepare for it by cutting your portions in half during the rest of the day. "If you can save 300 to 500 calories before the party, that means you can eat more," White says. But don't go to the party starving. "Curb your appetite with two glasses of water and something with fiber, like a cup of baby carrots with hummus, so you won't be ravenous when you head out the door."

2

HIT THE VEGGIE PLATTER

Appetizers are a waist-wrecker at parties because they're usually high in calories, drizzled in some kind of sauce, and so small that you can mindlessly pack away a half dozen before you've even said hello to the hosts. Stay away from the starchy stuff and load up your plate with veggies—they'll help keep your calories down and keep you full. "Many of these parties are held late at night, and you don't want to load up on carbohydrates then, anyway," White says.

3

PICK PROTEIN OVER PASTA

The protein station is also an area you'll want to hover around. Lettuce wraps, turkey slices, or other meat appetizers are good options because they'll keep you full and take longer to digest than muffins and breads.

4
SELECT YOUR SIN

"I always recommend if you're going to indulge in alcohol, don't indulge in food, or if you're going to indulge in food, don't indulge in alcohol," White says. "Pick your vice and stick with it—and try to keep it in moderation." And if you do choose to imbibe, try to drink one glass of water in between the alcoholic stuff. "That will slow you down, and keep you hydrated for the next day," White says.

5
TALK MORE, EAT LESS

The whole point of a party is to catch up with people, so spend more time chatting and less time chewing. At the dinner table, take a few bites then strike up a conversation with the person sitting next to you (please swallow first). Another trick is to match your partner or the person you're talking with, bite for bite. A British study found fast-eating men were 84 percent more likely to be overweight than slower eaters.

6
SHAKE UP YOUR CHEAT DAYS

White says he believes one cheat day a week is good for the body and mind. If you usually cheat on Sunday but have a party on Thursday, shift your schedule so you can eat guilt-free midweek.

7
WAKE UP TO YOGURT

The best way to recover from a holiday meal? Get right back on the horse. "Continue with your regular diet and exercise schedule, and let the previous day go," White says. "Start the next morning with a glass of water and something light, like fruit and yogurt, to detox the body. Then continue to eat light for the rest of the next day."

8
BURN IT OFF

Though there are many tricks and tips for losing weight, packing on the pounds comes down to simple math: Consume more than you burn off, and you'll gain weight. Sadly, increasing your exercise workload isn't an effective way to cancel out chronic binging, during the holidays or any time of the year.

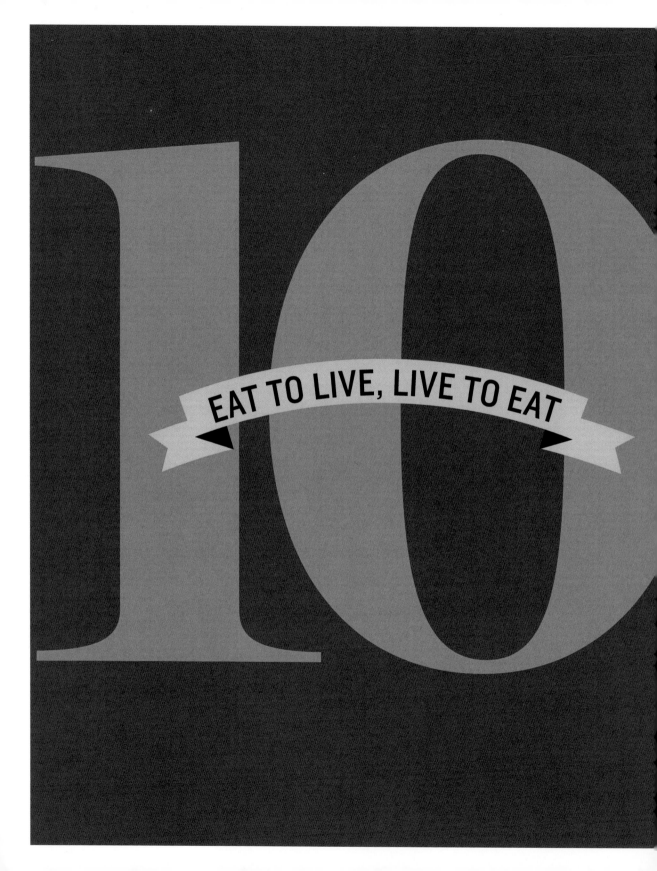

IO

EAT TO LIVE, LIVE TO EAT

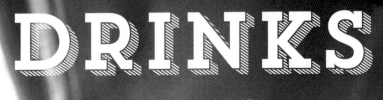

DRINKS

A guide to imbibing.

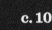

p. 266   c. 10

THE RULES *of* A DECENT HOME BAR

As your tastes evolve throughout your life, you might find this list charmingly minimalist. But everyone has to start their home bar somewhere. Before you get fancy, master the fundamentals.

RULE Nº.

1

ALWAYS STOCK THESE BOTTLES

CLEAR LIQUOR:
VODKA

Triple-distilled vodka ensures a smooth drink with good flavor balance. Buy: Grey Goose or Smirnoff.

GIN

It's a great base for spring and summer drinks. The best have a heady, floral aroma. Buy: Anchor Genevieve.

RUM

Opt for a sugarcane rum. It's well-balanced, but not too sweet. Buy: Appleton Estate Reserve.

WHISKEY

Use a smooth American brand to make Manhattans and Old Fashioneds. Buy: Jack Daniel's.

THE EXTRAS:
ANGOSTURA BITTERS

Add a few dashes of this aromatic concentration to drinks to add a layer of flavor.

VERMOUTH

Use the red variety in bourbon, whiskey, or scotch cocktails, and white with vodka or gin. Try either from Dolin Vermouth de Chambery.

MIXERS

Opt for fresh juices when possible, but canned ones work too. Try orange, grapefruit, or cranberry.

SIMPLE SYRUP: mix equal parts sugar and water; stir together until dissolved. Use for a Tom Collins, Hemmingway Daiquiri, French 75, or a Highline cocktail.

RULE Nº.

2 | SCORE THIS HARDWARE

A SMALL BUT powerful arsenal of tools will ensure there's never a cocktail challenge you can't solve. Find a great selection at cocktailkingdom.com and barsupplies.com.

JIGGER
For accurate measuring, don't eyeball it. Pick up a double jigger.

PARING KNIFE
Use to quickly slice garnishes without whipping out a chef's knife.

MIXING GLASS
For stirring rather than shaking, pick a mixing glass.

COCKTAIL SHAKER
Score a sturdy, stylish version of this drinks essential. Trust us, you'll be giving it a workout for years.

BAR SPOON
A teardrop bar spoon makes quick work of stirred drinks.

MUDDLER
A flat-headed steel muddler with a plastic top gives just the right amount of weight to your crushing tasks.

JULEP STRAINER
Clamp this tool over your shaker to free your drinks from pulp with ease.

CHANNEL KNIFE
The Tovolo Standz zester and channel knife makes pro-style citrus-peel twists simple.

WINE KEY
Don't go with one of those overblown bottle openers. The Victorinox lever corkscrew is simple and dependable.

3 | STOCK THIS GLASSWARE

THE SUPERSIZING OF the American diet has done more than threaten our waistlines. It's also wrecked our cocktails. "It's absurd. The cocktail glasses commonly sold today range from 7 to 13 ounces, even though the traditional recipes for drinks like the martini call for no more than 5 ounces of liquid," says Jason Wilson, author of *Boozehound*. He recommends finding classic glassware at bar- and restaurant-supply stores or yard sales.

 4½-ounce cocktail (aka martini) glasses

6- to 8-ounce Old-Fashioned or rocks glasses

10-ounce tall, slender highball glasses

 2-ounce cordial/shot glasses

RULE N°.

4 | MASTER THE MOVES

Concoct flawless cocktails by mastering these techniques with Jim Meehan, author of *The PDT Cocktail Book*.

THE STIR

THE TECHNIQUE Plunge the spoon three-quarters of the way into the glass with its back pressed against the side. Stir swiftly but smoothly for 8 to 12 seconds; move ice as one solid mass. Strain your drink into a chilled glass.

USE IT FOR Drinks prepared with spirits and fortified wines. Examples: martini, Negroni, Manhattan

THE TWIST

THE TECHNIQUE Position your hands over a cocktail glass to capture the citrus oils. Insert a channel knife's tooth-shaped notch into the fruit below the knob on the stem end. Press the knife firmly against the peel (without piercing the flesh), moving across and around the fruit, spacing each ring about ½" from the last one. Wrap the twist into a spiral around a straw; plop it into your finished drink.

USE IT FOR Citrus-based spirits or liqueurs, such as flavored vodka, gin, or triple sec. Examples: margarita, martini, Sazerac

THE SHAKE

THE TECHNIQUE Pour the liquid ingredients into the shaker; add about 2 cups of ice just before closing and shaking vigorously. "A lazy shake would only add undesirably large bubbles," says Meehan. A shake that lasts 8 to 12 seconds is ideal. "Shaking too long overdilutes the drink," Meehan says. Immediately strain into a chilled glass.

USE IT FOR Any drinks you prepare with citrus juice, egg whites, or cream (since they're meant to be cloudy). Examples: daiquiri, margarita, sidecar, pisco sour

CHEERS TO YOUR HEALTH
The medicinal value of a good drink.

Have you had your shots? During a 5-year period, lifetime alcohol abstainers were 19 percent more likely to die than regular drinkers—defined as people having one or two drinks, three or more days a week, say Virginia Tech University researchers. Those who never touched the bottle were also roughly 56 percent more likely to experience coronary heart disease than regular drinkers, found the scientists, who crunched data from a government survey of nearly half a million Americans. More reasons to drink to your health—in moderation, of course.

WHY BEER IS HEALTHY

Beer is just as good for your heart as red wine, according to an analysis of 18 studies on alcohol consumption. "After dissecting the effects of alcohol in wine and beer, the two beverages appeared to be quite comparable," explains Giovanni de Gaetano, M.D., Ph.D., director of Laboratory di Ricerca, where the study was conducted.

WHY WINE IS HEALTHY

In a recent Mount Sinai School of Medicine study on mice, polyphenols found in grapes were shown to decrease amyloid beta*56, a peptide associated with Alzheimer's. This is the first study to show that grape-derived polyphenols can reduce this peptide, possibly decreasing your risk of the disease.

WHY LIQUOR IS HEALTHY

A study, published in *Consciousness and Cognition*, included 40 men who watched a movie while they were asked to complete verbal puzzles. Half of the men were given enough of a vodka and cran- berry juice drink to get their blood alcohol content to .075— just below the legal limit of 0.08—while the other half were sober. The results? The buzzed guys solved problems faster than the sober ones—taking an average of 11.5 seconds versus 15.2—and out of 20 problems, correctly solved nine versus six for the sober set.

10 OLD-SCHOOL DRINKS

Every Man Must Know

1
MANHATTAN

This throwback cocktail has a bite of
bitters and a fiery whiskey finish.

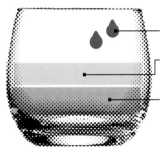

**2 to 4 dashes
Angostura bitters**

**1 ounce sweet
vermouth,**
like Noilly Prat

2 ounces bourbon

Pour the vermouth into a medium mixing glass.
Add the bourbon and bitters. Add ice and stir for
at least 20 seconds. Pour through a julep strainer
and into a chilled rocks or cocktail glass.

PER DRINK: 198 calories

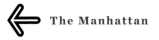
The Manhattan

2
BLOODY MARY

This is the ultimate brunch cocktail.
Make a pitcher for the crowd.

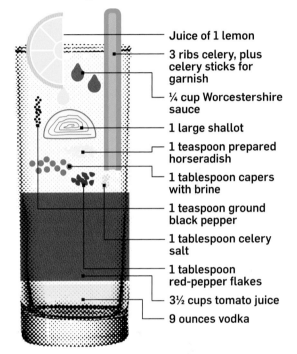

Juice of 1 lemon

**3 ribs celery, plus
celery sticks for
garnish**

**¼ cup Worcestershire
sauce**

1 large shallot

**1 teaspoon prepared
horseradish**

**1 tablespoon capers
with brine**

**1 teaspoon ground
black pepper**

**1 tablespoon celery
salt**

**1 tablespoon
red-pepper flakes**

3½ cups tomato juice

9 ounces vodka

In a blender, combine the celery, shallot,
horseradish, and capers and pulse until pureed.
Add the lemon juice, Worcestershire, and spices
and pulse briefly to combine.

Transfer the mixture to a pitcher and stir in the
tomato juice. Refrigerate the mix overnight.

To serve, run the chilled mixture through a
strainer and then pour it into 6 glasses. Add
about 1½ ounces vodka to each glass, along with
a cleaned and trimmed celery stick.

SERVES 6 // PER DRINK: 153 calories

3

HOT TODDY

There's nothing better than coming home after a long, cold day and warming up with one of these.

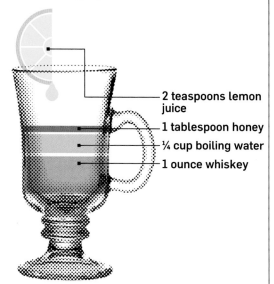

2 teaspoons lemon juice

1 tablespoon honey

¼ cup boiling water

1 ounce whiskey

Combine the whiskey, honey, and lemon juice in a glass mug. Top off with hot water, stir, and sip.

PER DRINK: 164 calories

4

OLD-FASHIONED

Appreciate the good ol' days with the drink that honors them.

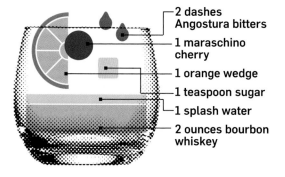

2 dashes Angostura bitters

1 maraschino cherry

1 orange wedge

1 teaspoon sugar

1 splash water

2 ounces bourbon whiskey

Mix the sugar, water and bitters in an Old-Fashioned glass. Muddle into a paste using a muddler or the back end of a spoon. Pour in the bourbon, fill with ice cubes, and stir. Drop in a cherry and an orange wedge.

PER DRINK: 159 calories

5

SAZERAC

This whiskey-based New Orleans
drink comes spiked with absinthe
and bitters.

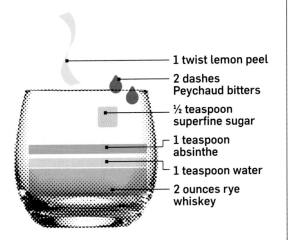

- 1 twist lemon peel
- 2 dashes Peychaud bitters
- ½ teaspoon superfine sugar
- 1 teaspoon absinthe
- 1 teaspoon water
- 2 ounces rye whiskey

Pour the absinthe into a glass and swirl around to
coat the glass; discard any excess. Add the sugar,
bitters, and water to the glass and muddle with
the back of a teaspoon. Almost fill the glass with
ice cubes. Pour the whiskey over the ice cubes
and add a twist of lemon peel.

PER DRINK: 143 calories

6

TOM COLLINS

Straightforward. Unpretentious.
Slightly sour. Just sweet enough.

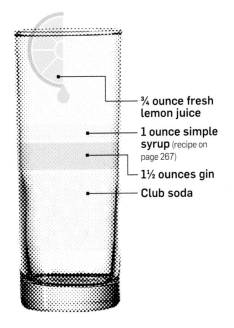

- ¾ ounce fresh lemon juice
- 1 ounce simple syrup (recipe on page 267)
- 1½ ounces gin
- Club soda

Shake the first three ingredients with ice and
strain into a cocktail glass. Top with club soda.

PER DRINK: 115 calories

7

MARGARITA

A real margarita doesn't involve a blender and, as long as your ingredients are made from the good stuff, you don't need a salt lick around the rim or fruit salad stuffed into the glass, either.

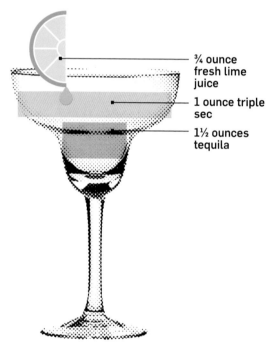

¾ ounce fresh lime juice

1 ounce triple sec

1½ ounces tequila

Shake these ingredients with ice and strain into a cocktail glass.

PER DRINK: 237 calories

8

NEGRONI

This simple drink contains just three ingredients, but packs a complexity that complicated cocktails can't match.

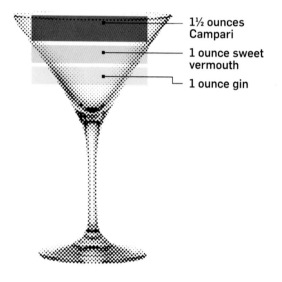

1½ ounces Campari

1 ounce sweet vermouth

1 ounce gin

Pour these ingredients into a cocktail glass with some crushed ice and give it a stir.

PER DRINK: 230 calories

9

MARTINI

Everybody wants to be Bond, but nobody gets it right—not even 007. The best martinis are stirred, not shaken.

10

WHISKEY SOUR

This mix can make even bottom-shelf whiskey taste like the good stuff.

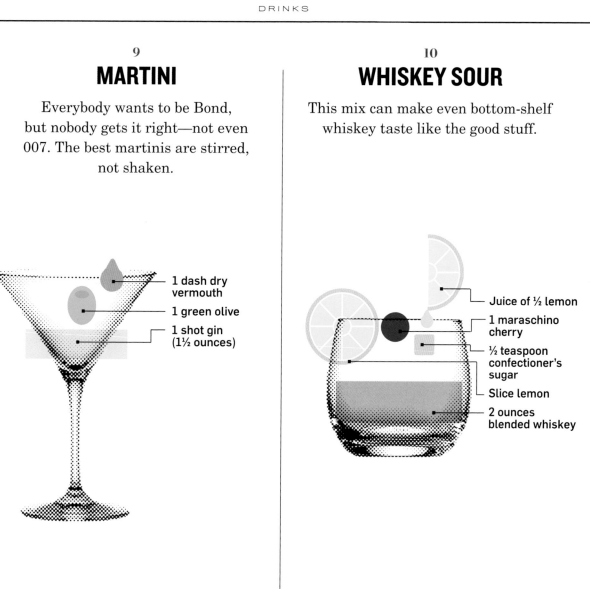

1 dash dry vermouth

1 green olive

1 shot gin (1½ ounces)

Juice of ½ lemon

1 maraschino cherry

½ teaspoon confectioner's sugar

Slice lemon

2 ounces blended whiskey

Chill the gin and vermouth over ice in a mixing glass. Then pour it into a frosted martini glass. Garnish with a green olive.

PER DRINK: 109 calories

Shake the whiskey, lemon juice, and sugar with ice and strain into a whiskey sour glass. Garnish with the lemon slice and top with the cherry.

PER DRINK: 150 calories

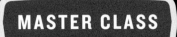

10 NEW-SCHOOL DRINKS
Every Man Must Know

1

HEMINGWAY DAIQUIRI

It's named after the lime concoction Papa drank, and it's far less fussy than the frozen slushy variety.

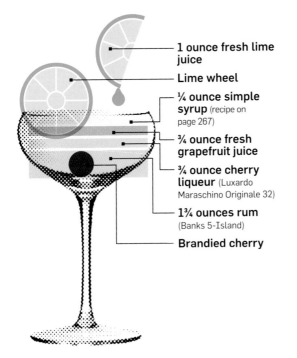

- **1 ounce fresh lime juice**
- **Lime wheel**
- **¼ ounce simple syrup** (recipe on page 267)
- **¾ ounce fresh grapefruit juice**
- **¾ ounce cherry liqueur** (Luxardo Maraschino Originale 32)
- **1¾ ounces rum** (Banks 5-Island)
- **Brandied cherry**

Shake with ice and strain into a chilled coupe glass. Garnish with a lime wheel speared with a brandied cherry.

PER DRINK: 215 calories

 The Hemingway Daiquiri

2

MEXICAN SUMMER SMASH COCKTAIL

In this citrusy highball, sweetness comes from agave nectar (with its low glycemic index and gentle effect on your blood sugar) and fresh fruit.

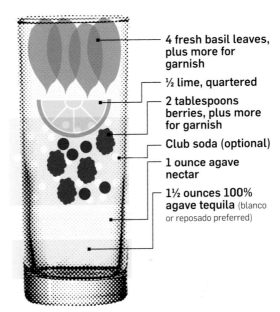

- **4 fresh basil leaves,** plus more for garnish
- **½ lime, quartered**
- **2 tablespoons berries,** plus more for garnish
- **Club soda (optional)**
- **1 ounce agave nectar**
- **1½ ounces 100% agave tequila** (blanco or reposado preferred)

In a mixing glass, combine the basil, lime quarters, berries, and agave nectar. Muddle to extract the juices from all the fruit. Add the tequila and ice, and shake vigorously. Pour into a Collins glass and garnish with fresh berries and basil. If you like a bit of fizz in your cocktails (and want to stretch them a bit further), top with an ounce or two of club soda.

PER DRINK: 261 calories

2

WATERMELON DAIQUIRI

It's not as frilly as you think. The watermelon, cut into cubes and frozen, stands in for ice cubes, delivering a dose of sweetness that balances out the rum.

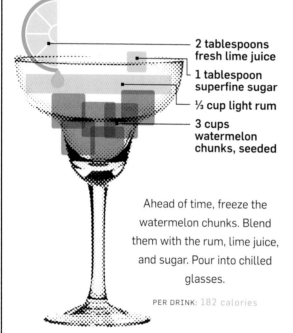

- 2 tablespoons fresh lime juice
- 1 tablespoon superfine sugar
- ⅓ cup light rum
- 3 cups watermelon chunks, seeded

Ahead of time, freeze the watermelon chunks. Blend them with the rum, lime juice, and sugar. Pour into chilled glasses.

PER DRINK: 182 calories

4

FRENCH 75

This champagne-based drink makes a great aperitif. Traditionally served in a Collins glass, it also looks romantic in a flute. If you don't like gin, use brandy, Cognac, or Calvados.

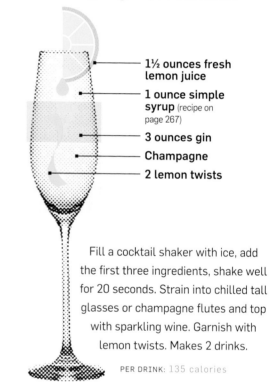

- 1½ ounces fresh lemon juice
- 1 ounce simple syrup (recipe on page 267)
- 3 ounces gin
- Champagne
- 2 lemon twists

Fill a cocktail shaker with ice, add the first three ingredients, shake well for 20 seconds. Strain into chilled tall glasses or champagne flutes and top with sparkling wine. Garnish with lemon twists. Makes 2 drinks.

PER DRINK: 135 calories

HOW TO POUR CHAMPAGNE

TEMPERATURE Chill the bottle to 39°F. (Just check your fridge thermometer.) That's the temperature at which champagne retains the most bubbles. And that's what it's all about.

5

GIN RICKEY

If you're a gin and tonic drinker looking to cut calories, try a Gin Rickey.
Club soda actually has less sugar
than tonic water.

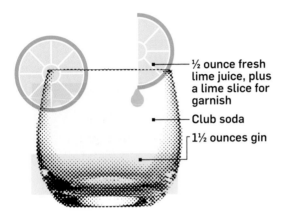

½ ounce fresh
lime juice, plus
a lime slice for
garnish

Club soda

1½ ounces gin

Combine the gin and lime juice in an ice-filled
rocks glass; top up with club soda and garnish
with a slice of lime.

PER DRINK: 100 calories

6

PRESBYTERIAN

It's the more sophisticated (and less
sweet) cousin of the whiskey sour. Sip
if you're looking for something on the
lighter side.

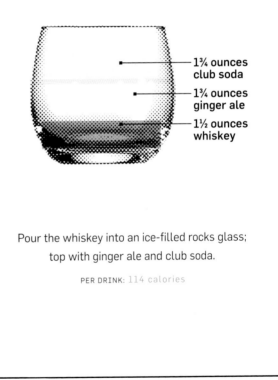

1¾ ounces
club soda

1¾ ounces
ginger ale

1½ ounces
whiskey

Pour the whiskey into an ice-filled rocks glass;
top with ginger ale and club soda.

PER DRINK: 114 calories

ANGLE Hold the flute at a 45-degree angle,
resting the bottom edge on a table, so the
champagne can slide in gently. Don't pour it into
an upright glass; this destroys the bubbles.

TOUCH For a smooth pour with minimal bubble
loss, touch the bottle to the glass.

7

BLOOD & SAND

It's deep red because it's colored with
a touch of cherry liqueur, which also
tempers the fire of Scotch.

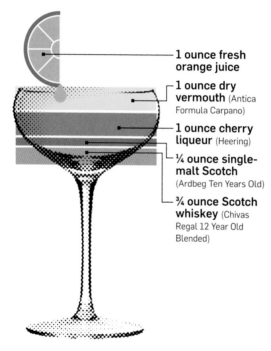

1 ounce fresh
orange juice

1 ounce dry
vermouth (Antica
Formula Carpano)

1 ounce cherry
liqueur (Heering)

¼ ounce single-
malt Scotch
(Ardbeg Ten Years Old)

¾ ounce Scotch
whiskey (Chivas
Regal 12 Year Old
Blended)

Shake with ice and strain into a
chilled coupe glass.

PER DRINK: 200 calories

8

TEQUILA GO-TO

Far more refreshing than any
mass-produced, fruit-tinged beer,
this drink pulls its crisp flavors from
fresh vegetables and herbs.

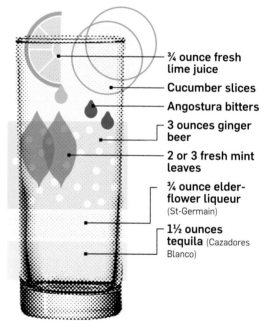

¾ ounce fresh
lime juice

Cucumber slices

Angostura bitters

3 ounces ginger
beer

2 or 3 fresh mint
leaves

¾ ounce elder-
flower liqueur
(St-Germain)

1½ ounces
tequila (Cazadores
Blanco)

Add the tequila, elderflower liqueur, lime juice,
cucumber slices, and mint leaves to a shaker.
Add ice, shake briefly, and dump into a
Collins glass. Top up with ginger beer and
garnish with a dash of bitters.

PER DRINK: 205 calories

9
GINGER SMASH

Hit your cocktails with a slug or two of "mixer" and you're adding needless corn syrups and additives. Fresh fruit and real sugar work just fine, as evidenced in this drink, also tinged with the sharp taste of ginger.

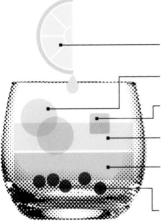

- ¾ ounce fresh lemon juice
- A couple of slices of fresh ginger
- 1½ teaspoons superfine sugar
- 1½ ounces gin (Plymouth)
- 1½ ounces apple liqueur (Berentzen Apfelkorn)
- 5 or 6 fresh cranberries

In an Old-Fashioned glass, use a muddler or bar spoon to lightly pound the ginger—no need to pulverize. Add the cranberries and sugar and muddle again. Add the gin, apple liqueur, and lemon juice. Then fill the glass with ice and pour the contents into a shaker. Shake briefly and pour everything back into the glass.

PER DRINK: 268 calories

10
HIGH LINE COCKTAIL

For an alternative to the hot toddy, enjoy this spicy cocktail, created by bartender Markus Tschuschnig of Morimoto in New York City.

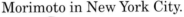
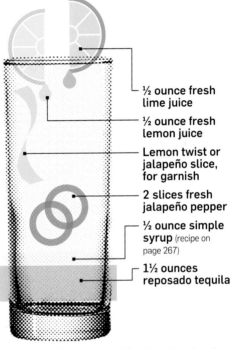

- ½ ounce fresh lime juice
- ½ ounce fresh lemon juice
- Lemon twist or jalapeño slice, for garnish
- 2 slices fresh jalapeño pepper
- ½ ounce simple syrup (recipe on page 267)
- 1½ ounces reposado tequila

In a cocktail shaker, muddle the jalapeño slices with the simple syrup. Add the other ingredients and top up the shaker with ice. Shake, and then pour into an ice-filled Collins glass. Garnish with a lemon twist or jalapeño slice.

PER DRINK: 121 calories

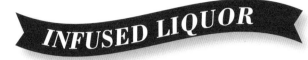

We've all seen the shelf-buckling load
of fruit-flavored spirits at the liquor store. The
problem is, few of those bottles contain true infusions.
They're flavored spirits, and "flavored" usually
means a combination of sugar, colorings, and
fake-tasting additives. "But when you and I infuse
something, we know exactly what's in it," says
Marcus Samuelsson, the owner of New York City's
Red Rooster Harlem and Ginny's Supper Club
restaurants. "Pick the formula that speaks to you,
start your infusion, and your house cocktails will
never be the same again."

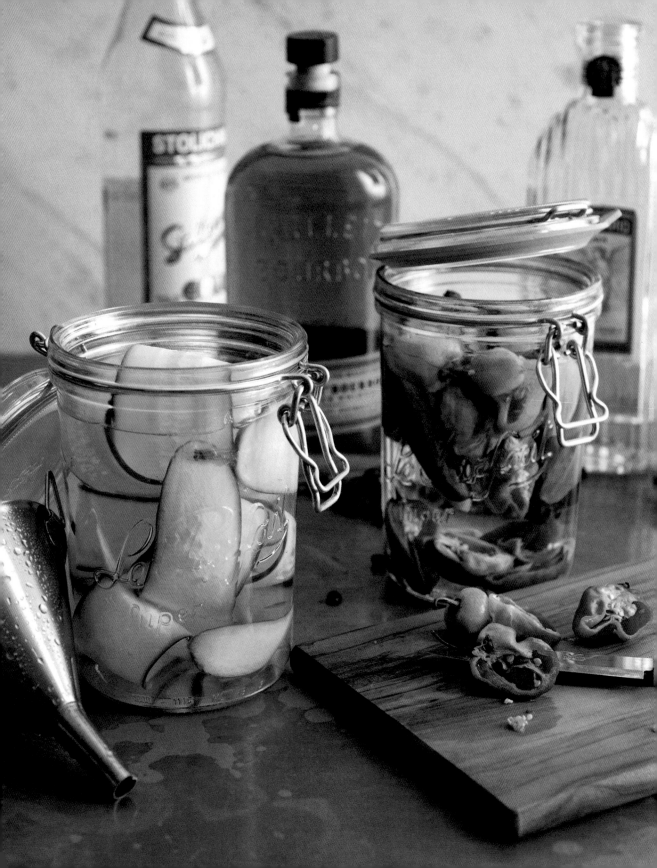

INFUSED LIQUOR

YOU'LL NEED:

WIDE-MOUTH JARS OR BOTTLES (FOR
THE INFUSION) // SIEVE // ASSORTED
RESEALABLE GLASS BOTTLES OR FLASKS
(FOR THE FINISHED PRODUCT) // FUNNEL

1 USE CHEAP BOOZE

You can infuse any spirit you like, but there's no need to waste money on the expensive stuff. Most of the flavor will come from the infusion, so the nuances of, say, a 12-year-old whiskey will be lost to the ingredients you add. For each dose that you add of the flavoring ingredients, you'll need a fifth of vodka, reposado tequila, or bourbon.

2 CHOOSE YOUR VESSEL

Pour your booze into a wide-mouth jar or bottle, leaving enough space for the flavorings. (If using a bottle, make sure your flavorings fit through the neck.)

3 PAIR ALCOHOL FLAVORING

BOURBON

FIGS
Puree ½ cup dried, stemmed figs (pitted prunes work too) with a splash of bourbon in a food processor.

VODKA

CUCUMBER
Peel 1 large cucumber (the peel can make the infusion bitter) and cut it into thick slices.

TEQUILA

PINEAPPLE
Peel, core, and cut up a ripe pineapple to yield 1 cup of chunks, or use canned pineapple chunks in juice.

PEANUTS

Roast 1 cup salted or unsalted peanuts at 350°F for 12 minutes and then dump them immediately into the jar or bottle.

COFFEE

Add ½ cup of your favorite roasted whole coffee beans.

FENNEL AND CARAWAY

Pan-toast 2 tablespoons caraway seeds in a dry skillet until fragrant, and thinly slice one-third of a fennel bulb.

CITRUS

Cut away the peel of 2 or 3 oranges, grapefruits, lemons, and/or limes (1 to 2 if they're large). Then lightly mash the fruit, tossing any seeds.

CHILES

Quarter 2 or 3 fresh serrano, jalapeño, or habanero chiles to expose the spicy ribs and seeds.

LEMONGRASS AND GINGER

Add ¼ cup chopped fresh ginger and 2 lemongrass stalks, tough outer leaves removed, sliced into rings.

4 STEEP THE CONCOCTION

A full-flavored extraction can take up to 2 weeks to create, but taste the liquor along the way to be sure: Chile infusions are done in 2 to 3 days, juicier fruits take longer, and bigger chunks of aromatics like ginger require the most time. When the liquor achieves the right flavor level, strain the infusion and then funnel it into a clean bottle or jar.

5 USE IT

"Infused spirits make great gifts for guys," says Samuelsson. "Funnel it into a flask, put a buddy's name on it, and give it to him just like that. It's unique and it shows you thought about him."

KEEP YOUR SPIRITS STRAIGHT

If you have multiple infusions going on, slap labels on your jars with the date and the flavorings for each one.

COCKTAIL MATRIX

A
CHOOSE YOUR BASE SPIRIT

Start by picking a foundation liquor, adding 1½ to 3 ounces to your mixing glass. (Never build a cocktail over ice—you'll end up with an overly diluted drink.) As you pour, give your base spirit a sniff and start thinking about the flavors that would work best with it.

B
ADD A SWEET COMPONENT

Bartenders use sugar the way chefs use salt—as an essential seasoning. Sugar or sugary liqueurs enhance the liquor, soothe the alcohol burn, and add a layer of flavor. Depending on the drink, you'll want anywhere from a cube of sugar to an ounce of sweet liqueur.

C
ADD A BITTER (OR ACIDIC) COMPONENT

Infuse dimension into your cocktail by contrasting sweetness with bitterness or acid or both. A good guideline for citrus is 1 part sour to 1¼ parts sweet. With bitters, you need only a few dashes. Then shake or stir to create your cocktail.

D
GARNISH WITH STYLE

An easy rule of thumb: If it's a flavor or a fresh ingredient that's already in your drink, it makes a great garnish. A fresh lemon twist complements the citrus botanicals in a gin martini. Another route? Think about contrast— a briny olive in your martini will be a salty foil for the gin's juniper.

Classic drinks contain just a few basic elements.
Learn the principles of mixology and craft your own.

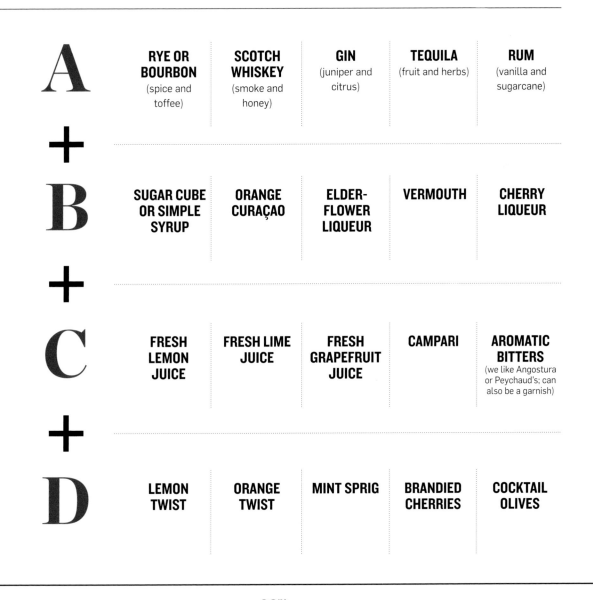

A

RYE OR BOURBON (spice and toffee)	SCOTCH WHISKEY (smoke and honey)	GIN (juniper and citrus)	TEQUILA (fruit and herbs)	RUM (vanilla and sugarcane)

+

B

SUGAR CUBE OR SIMPLE SYRUP	ORANGE CURAÇAO	ELDER-FLOWER LIQUEUR	VERMOUTH	CHERRY LIQUEUR

+

C

FRESH LEMON JUICE	FRESH LIME JUICE	FRESH GRAPEFRUIT JUICE	CAMPARI	AROMATIC BITTERS (we like Angostura or Peychaud's; can also be a garnish)

+

D

LEMON TWIST	ORANGE TWIST	MINT SPRIG	BRANDIED CHERRIES	COCKTAIL OLIVES

Best Beers

Beer makes you feel good. You knew that. But you don't realize just how good. Recent research has revealed bioactive compounds in beer that battle cancer, boost your metabolism, and more. And these benefits come on top of the oft-touted upsides of moderate alcohol intake: clot prevention, cleaner arteries, and reduced stress. We set out with a stack of studies, a panel of parched testers, and a full fridge to find the best-tasting, healthiest brews available. Enjoy.

Best Hops Delivery Vehicle
AVERY MAHARAJA IMPERIAL INDIA PALE ALE

Hops help cut the sweetness in a beer, delivering a crisp citrus-and-pine kick to the back of your tongue. But the cone-shaped hops flower is more than just a flavor savior. Researchers have shown that it's also a significant source of cholesterol-lowering, cancer-fighting, and virus-killing compounds called polyphenols. What's more, "Just one 12-ounce beer a day decreased fibrinogen, a clotting factor, and increased albumin, which is very important for protein metabolism," says Shela Gorinstein, Ph.D., a researcher at Jerusalem's Hebrew University and the author of a 2007 study on the bioactivity of beer. In our taste test, the winner was a smooth, fruity India Pale Ale (IPA) brewed with 8 pounds of hops per barrel. It boasts 80 times the hops of a mass-market lager.

RUNNER-UP: **Southern Tier Unearthly IPA**
ALSO TRY: North Coast Brewing Red Seal Ale, Harpoon IPA, Sierra Nevada Pale Ale, Stone IPA, Two Hearted Ale

Best Low-Cal Beer
BEAMISH IRISH STOUT

The typical low-cal beer is run through a deflavorizing machine on its way to the bottle. "Most of the calories come from the alcohol content and whatever residual sugars may be left after fermentation," says Garrett Oliver, brewmaster at the Brooklyn Brewery. We sought a brew that would go easy on the waistline without disappointing the palate. Darker beers have a major advantage here: They're relatively low in alcohol and have thick, creamy, smoky finishes. When the cans were emptied, Beamish stood tall. It contains about 130 calories per 12-ounce can, but with a full flavor and sturdy dark-chocolate notes.

RUNNER-UP: **New Belgium Skinny Dip**
ALSO TRY: Sam Adams Light, Guinness Draught, Sprecher Micro-Light Ale, Mahr's Bräu Leicht, Shiner Light

Best Organic Beer
WOLAVER'S INDIA PALE ALE

The German Beer Purity Law of 1516 restricted "true" beer to three ingredients: water, barley, and hops. Today's megabrewery beers are anything but pure. A 2003 FDA study found that 27 percent of barley and 32 percent of nonorganic wheat products carried pesticide residues. What's worse, a loophole in the USDA organic-certification standard allows pesticide-grown hops. Our winner, an IPA with a pleasant aftertaste, is made with wheat from organic farms near the brewer's Vermont facility. "We track every detail of every organic ingredient," says Max Oswald, a Wolaver's spokesman.

RUNNER-UP: **Butte Creek Brewing Pilsner**
ALSO TRY: Peak Organic Amber, Dupont Foret, Old Plowshare Stout, Orlio IPA, Samuel Smith's Organic Ale

Best Alterna-Brew
HE'BREW ORIGIN POMEGRANATE ALE

Novelty beers can be cloying—you can't drink more than one—and few of the added ingredients pack health benefits. In our taste test, our top pick featured the antioxidant-laden superfruit pomegranate, shown to combat cancer and lower your risk of Alzheimer's and heart disease. In a 2006 UCLA study, for example, men who drank a glass of pomegranate juice every day reduced prostate-cancer cell growth by 12 percent. Brewers dump more than 150 gallons of pomegranate juice into every batch (equivalent to 10,000 pomegranates, or half of a fruit per bottle), giving the final product a raspberry-like flavor that allows the malt and hops to come through.

RUNNER-UP: **Dogfish Head Black & Blue**
ALSO TRY: Barons Black Wattle Ale, Rogue Juniper Pale Ale, Lindemans Framboise, Kelpie Seaweed Ale

Best Bottle-Conditioned Beer
BROOKLYN BREWERY LOCAL I

With bottle-conditioned beers, brewer's yeast is added right before the bottle is closed, reigniting the fermentation process. The result: deeper flavors, extra effervescence, and, it turns out, many health benefits—the yeast is a rich source of B-complex vitamins, protein, and minerals such as chromium. "German doctors used to prescribe bottle-conditioned wheat beer to patients with vitamin deficiencies," says Oliver. As a probiotic organism, yeast helps your body break down nutrients, regulates your digestive system, maintains your nervous system, and even helps modulate blood-sugar levels. Oliver's Local 1 won with a balanced blend of spices and subtle malt flavors. Bonus: Its brewmaster uses twice the yeast.

RUNNER-UP: **Southampton Grand Cru**
ALSO TRY: Ommegang Hennepin, Tripel Karmaliet, Franziskaner Hefe-Weisse Hell, Allagash White, La Fin du Monde

Best Dark Malt
TRAPPISTES ROCHEFORT 8

The smooth, deep finish of a dark malt develops during the same high-temperature roasting process that fuels the formation of antioxidants. "Dark beers are loaded with them," says Joe Vinson, Ph.D., a researcher at the University of Scranton. Vinson showed in a 2003 study that stouts, porters, and browns contain more than twice the antioxidants of lagers, on average. What's more, "The antioxidants in beer are better at reacting with toxic free radicals than the ones in antioxidant vitamin pills." The Rochefort's creamy cocoa and caramel notes won us over.

RUNNER-UP: **Goose Island Bourbon County Stout**
ALSO TRY: Alaskan Smoked Porter, Samuel Smith's Nut Brown, Anchor Porter, Shakespeare Stout, Ayinger Celebrator

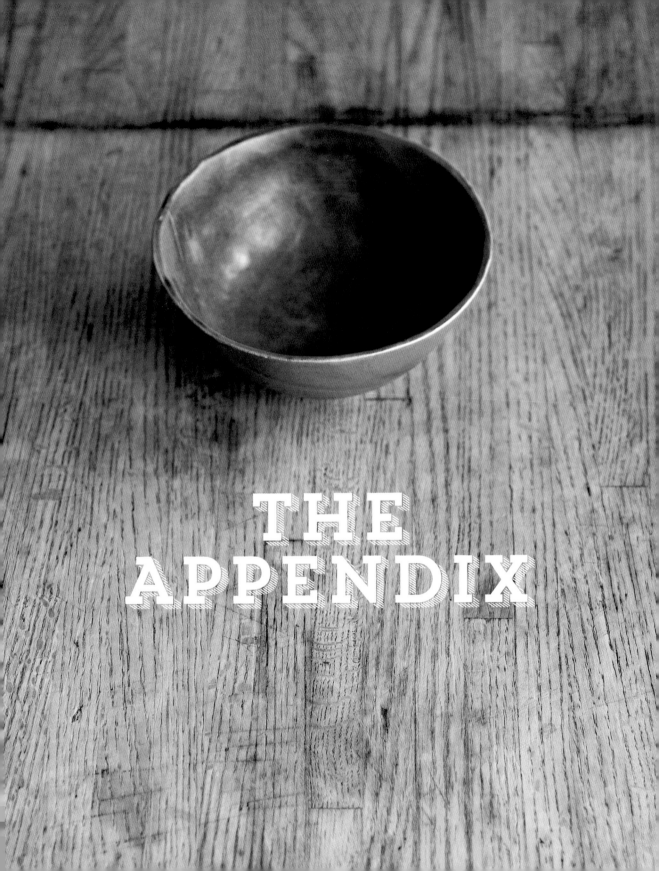

THE
APPENDIX

NUTRITIONAL VALUES OF COMMON FOODS

	VITAMIN A (MCG)	VITAMIN B$_1$ (THIAMIN) (MG)	VITAMIN B$_6$ (MG)	FOLATE (MCG)	VITAMIN C (MG)
RDA (men/women)	**900/700**	**1.2/1.1**	**1.3/1.3**	**400/400**	**95/75**
Almonds (1 ounce)	0	0.05	0.03	11	0
Apple (1 medium)	8	0.02	0.06	4	6
Apricot (1)	67	0.01	0.02	3	3.50
Artichoke (1 medium)	0	0.10	0.15	87	15
Asparagus (1 medium spear)	12	0.02	0.01	8	1
Avocado (1)	122	0.20	0.60	124	16
Bacon (3 slices)	0	0.08	0.07	0.40	0
Bagel (4 inches)	0	0.15	0.05	20	0
Banana (1 medium)	7	0.04	0.40	24	10
Beans, baked (1 cup)	13	0.40	0.34	61	8
Beans, black (1 cup cooked)	1	0.40	0.12	256	0
Beans, kidney (1 cup cooked)	0	0.28	0.21	230	2
Beans, lima (½ cup cooked)	32	0.12	0.16	22	9
Beans, navy (1 cup cooked)	0.36	0.40	0.30	255	1.64
Beans, pinto (1 cup cooked)	0	0.17	0.16	294	1.37
Beans, refried (1 cup)	0	0.07	0.36	28	15
Beans, white (1 cup cooked)	0	0.20	0.17	145	0
Beef, ground lean (3 ounces)	0	0.06	0.24	7	0
Beer (12 ounces)	0	0.02	0.18	21	0
Beets (½ cup)	3	0.02	0.05	74	3
Blueberries (1 pint)	17	0.11	0.15	17	28
Bran, wheat (1 cup)	0	0.14	0.35	14	0
Bread, rye (1 slice)	0.26	0.14	0.02	35	0.13
Bread, white (1 slice)	0	0.11	0.02	28	0
Bread, whole grain (1 slice)	0	0.11	0.10	30	0.08
Breakfast sandwich, fast-food (bacon, egg, and cheese)	0	0.53	0.16	73	2
Brussels sprouts (½ cup)	60	0.08	0.14	47	48
Cake, coffee (1 piece)	20	0.10	0.03	27	0.11

VITAMIN E (MG)	CALCIUM (MG)	MAGNESIUM (MG)	POTASSIUM (MG)	SELENIUM (MCG)	ZINC (MG)	CALORIES
15/15	**1,000/1,000**	**420/320**	**4,700/4,700**	**55/55**	**11/8**	**–**
6	71	86	180	0	1	170
0.25	8	7	148	0	0.06	80
0.30	5	3.50	90	0.03	0.07	20
0.24	56	77	474	0.26	0.60	25
0.18	4	2	32	0.37	0.10	5
3	22	78	1,204	0.80	0.84	25
0.06	2	6	107	12	0.70	110
0.04	16	26	90	28	1	247
0.12	6	32	422	1	0.20	110
1.35	127	81	752	12	4	239
0.14	46	120	610	2	1.90	240
0.05	62	74	717	2	1.80	260
0.12	27	63	485	1.70	0.70	229
0.73	127	107	670	11	1.90	255
1.61	72	70	495	19	1.70	245
0	88	83	675	3	3	240
1.74	161	113	1,004	2.30	2.50	249
0.15	7	19	265	0	4	185
0	18	21	89	2.50	0.04	153
0.03	111	16	221	0.5	0.24	29
1.65	17	17	223	0.3	0.50	165
0.54	26	220	426	28	3	120
0.11	23	13	53	10	0.36	83
0.06	38	6	25	4.30	0.20	67
0.09	24	14	53	8	0.30	65
0.60	160	24	211	36.0	2	441
0.34	28	16	247	1.17	0.26	28
0.11	76	10	63	9	0.25	180

	VITAMIN A (MCG)	VITAMIN B₁ (THIAMIN) (MG)	VITAMIN B₆ (MG)	FOLATE (MCG)	VITAMIN C (MG)
RDA (men/women)	**900/700**	**1.2/1.1**	**1.3/1.3**	**400/400**	**95/75**
Cake, frosted (1 piece)	10	0.01	0.02	7	0.04
Canadian bacon (2 slices)	0	0.40	0.20	2	0
Candy, nonchocolate (1 package)	0	0	0	0	0
Cantaloupe (1 medium wedge)	345	0.04	0.07	21	37
Carrot (1)	734	0.04	0.08	12	4
Cauliflower (1 cup)	2	0.06	0.22	57	46
Celery (1 cup, strips)	55	0.03	0.10	45	4
Cereal, whole grain, with raisins (½ cup)	3	0.16	0.10	22	0.55
Cheddar cheese (1 slice)	75	0.01	0.2	5	0
Chef's salad with no dressing (1½ cups)	146	0.40	0.40	101	16
Cherries, sweet, raw (1 cup)	30	0.07	0.05	5.80	10
Chicken, skinless (½ breast)	4	0.04	0.32	2	0.71
Chickpeas (1 cup cooked)	4	0.19	0.22	282	2
Chili with beans (1 cup)	87	0.12	0.30	59	4
Chips, potato, light (1 ounce)	0	0.05	0.22	8	3.40
Chocolate (1.45 ounces)	20	0.05	0.01	5	0
Cinnamon bun (1)	0	0.12	0	17	0.06
Citrus fruits and frozen concentrate juices (12 ounces)	7	0.17	0.30	31	324
Clams, fried (¾ cup)	101	0.11	0.07	41	11.25
Coffee (1 cup)	0	0	0	5	0
Collards (1 cup cooked)	0.08	0.8	0.24	177	35
Cookie, chocolate chip (1)	0.04	0.01	0.01	0.90	0
Corn (1 cup)	0.26	0.06	0.16	115	12
Cottage cheese, low-fat (1 cup)	25	0.05	0.15	27	0
Crackers (12)	0	0.17	0	0	0
Cranberry juice cocktail (1 cup)	1	0.02	0.05	0	90
Cream cheese (1 tablespoon)	53	0	0	2	0
Cucumber with peel (½ cup)	10	0.01	0.02	7	2.76
Doughnut (1)	17	0.10	0.03	24	0.09
Egg, whole (1 large)	84	0.03	0.06	22	0
Eggplant (1 cup)	4	0.08	0.09	14	1
English muffin, whole wheat (1)	0.09	0.25	0.05	36	0
Fig bar cookies (2 bars)	3	0.05	0.02	11	0.10

VITAMIN E (MG)	CALCIUM (MG)	MAGNESIUM (MG)	POTASSIUM (MG)	SELENIUM (MCG)	ZINC (MG)	CALORIES
15/15	**1,000/1,000**	**420/320**	**4,700/4,700**	**55/55**	**11/8**	**–**
0	18	14	84	1.40	0.30	239
0.16	5	10	181	11	0.80	137
0	0	0	0	0	0	230
0.05	9	12	272	0.40	0.18	24
0.40	20	7	195	0.06	0.15	35
0.08	22	15	303	0.60	0.30	25
0.33	50	14	322	0.50	0.16	17
0.40	33	70	207	10	1	195
0.08	204	8	28	4	0.90	114
0	235	49	401	37	3	267
0.20	21	16	325	0.90	0.09	90
0.08	6.50	16	150	11	0.50	130
0.60	80	79	477	6	2.50	269
1.46	120	115	934	3	5	220
0.62	10	18	285	2	0.17	142
0.83	78	26	153	2	0.83	230
0.48	10	3.60	19	5	0.10	418
0.24	85	68	1,336	1	0.41	186
0	71	16	366	33	1.60	560
0.05	2	5	114	0	0.02	2
1.67	266	38	220	1	0.50	61
0.26	2.50	3	14	0	0.06	63
0.15	8	44	343	1.54	1.36	120
0.02	138	11	194	20	.86	180
0	28	12	48	2.40	0.20	155
0	8	5	46	0	0.18	137
0.04	12	1	17	0.40	0.10	51
0	7	6	75	0	0.10	8
0.90	21	9	60	4	0.30	230
0.50	25	5	63	15	0.50	74
0.40	6	11	122	0.10	0.12	35
0.26	101	21	106	17	0.61	134
0.21	20	9	66	1	0.12	111

	VITAMIN A (MCG)	VITAMIN B₁ (THIAMIN) (MG)	VITAMIN B₆ (MG)	FOLATE (MCG)	VITAMIN C (MG)
RDA (men/women)	**900/700**	**1.2/1.1**	**1.3/1.3**	**400/400**	**95/75**
Fish, white (1 fillet)	60	0.26	0.50	26	0
French fries (10)	0	0.07	0.16	8	6
Fruit, dried (1 ounce)	208	0.01	0.05	1.10	1
Fruit juice, unsweetened (1 cup)	0	0.02	0.06	35	40
Garlic (1 clove)	0	0	0.04	0.09	0.90
Graham cracker (1 large rectangular piece)	0	0.03	0.01	6	0
Granola bar (1)	2	0.06	0.02	6	0.22
Grape juice (1 cup)	1	0.07	0.16	8	0.25
Ham (1 slice)	0	0.20	0.10	1	0
Hamburger, fast-food, with condiments and vegetables (1)	4	0.30	0.12	52	2
Hot dog, fast-food (1)	0	0.44	0.09	85	0.09
Ice cream (1 serving)	6	0.03	0.04	11	0.46
Jam or preserves (1 tablespoon)	0.20	0.0	0	2	2
Kale (1 cup)	955	0.07	0.11	18	33
Ketchup (1 tablespoon)	7	0	0.02	2	2
Kiwifruit (1 medium)	3	0.02	0.07	19	70
Lasagna, meat (7 ounces)	61	0.19	0.20	16	12
Lentils (1 cup cooked)	4.75	0.33	0.35	358	0.22
Lettuce, iceberg (1 cup)	8	0.02	0.03	31	2
Lettuce, romaine (½ cup)	81	0.02	0.02	38	7
Liver, beef (3 ounces)	8,042	0.16	0.86	215	1.62
Lunchmeat, salami (3 slices)	0	0.10	0.08	0.34	0
Macaroni and cheese (8 ounces)	48	0.25	0	0	0
Meat loaf (1 slice)	20	0.10	0.14	12	0.62
Melon, honeydew (1 cup)	5	0.07	0.16	34	32
Milk, fat-free (1 cup)	5	0.10	0.10	12	2
Milk, soy (1 cup)	0	0.15	0.16	40	0
Muffin, blueberry (1)	13	0.10	0.01	42	0.63
Mushrooms (1 cup sliced)	0	0.09	0.10	12	2
Nachos with cheese (6–8)	170	0.20	0.20	12	1
Nectarine (1)	23	0.05	0.03	7	7
Oatmeal (1 cup)	0.12	0.12	0.10	13	0
Olives (1 tablespoon)	1.70	0	0	0	0
Onion rings (10 medium)	0.98	0.10	0.07	64	0.68
Oyster (1 medium)	4.20	0.01	0.01	1.40	0.51
Pancakes (2)	7.60	0.16	0.07	28	0.15

VITAMIN E (MG)	CALCIUM (MG)	MAGNESIUM (MG)	POTASSIUM (MG)	SELENIUM (MCG)	ZINC (MG)	CALORIES
15/15	**1,000/1,000**	**420/320**	**4,700/4,700**	**55/55**	**11/8**	–
0.39	51	65	625	25	2	168
0.12	4	11	211	0.20	0.20	100
0.31	11.82	11.13	226	0	0.14	69
0.20	160	9	154	0	0.20	117
0	5	0.75	12	0.40	0	4
0	3	4	19	1	0.10	59
0.05	15	24	82	4	0.50	117
0.62	23	25	334	0.25	0.13	154
0.32	2	5	94	6	0.50	30
0	126	23	251	20	2	512
.10	108	27	190	29	2	242
0	72	19	164	1.65	0.40	133
0	4	0.80	15	.40	0	56
1	180	23	417	1.17	0.23	39
0.20	3	3	57	0.04	0	15
1	26	13	237	0.15	0.10	50
0.94	220	41	372	28	3	318
2.97	37	71	731	5.54	2.51	230
0.02	11	4	84	0.28	0.10	8
0.04	9	4	69	0.10	0.06	5
0.43	5	18	300	31	4.50	162
0.05	1.34	2.86	63	4	0.54	150
0	102	0	111	0	0	415
0.10	43	22	295	0	4	231
0.04	11	18	403	1.24	0.15	61
0.10	301	27	406	5	1	83
0	80	60	440	3	0.90	100
0.47	32	9	70	6	0.30	158
0.10	5	10	355	8	0.70	15
0	311	63	196	18	2	296
1	8	12	273	0	0.23	70
0.26	19	51	175	0	1.43	150
0.14	7	0.30	0.67	0.08	0	10
0.39	86	19	152	3	0.41	370
0.12	6	7	22	9	13	41
0.65	96	15	133	10	0.30	173

	VITAMIN A (MCG)	VITAMIN B₁ (THIAMIN) (MG)	VITAMIN B₆ (MG)	FOLATE (MCG)	VITAMIN C (MG)
RDA (men/women)	**900/700**	**1.2/1.1**	**1.3/1.3**	**400/400**	**95/75**
Pasta with red sauce (4.5 ounces)	0	0.13	0.10	4	6
Peach (1 medium)	15	0.02	0.02	4	6
Peanut butter (2 tablespoons)	0	0.03	0.15	24	0
Peanuts (1 ounce)	0	0.12	0.07	41	0
Pear (1 medium)	1.60	0.02	0.05	12	7
Pepper, chile, raw (½ pepper)	21.6	0.03	0.23	10.35	65
Peppers, sweet (10 strips)	78	0.04	0.13	13	70
Pie, apple (1 piece)	37	0.03	0.04	32	4
Pizza, cheese (1 slice)	74	0.20	0.04	35	1
Pizza, vegetable (1 slice)	58	0.40	0.50	116	79
Plum (1)	21	0.03	0.05	1.45	6
Popcorn (1 cup)	0.80	0.02	0.02	2	0
Pork (3 ounces)	0	0.80	0.30	3	0
Potatoes, mashed (1 cup)	8.40	0.20	0.50	17	13
Potato salad (1 cup)	2.93	0.20	0.40	19	19
Potpie, chicken	256	0.30	0.20	41	2
Pretzels (10 twists)	0	0.30	0.07	103	0
Raisins (1.5 ounces)	0	0.05	0.08	1.28	2.30
Raspberries (10)	0.38	0.01	0.01	4	5
Rice, brown (1 cup)	0	0.20	0.30	8	0
Rice, white (1 cup)	0	0.03	0.15	5	0
Ricotta cheese, part skim (½ cup)	132	0.03	0.02	16	0
Salad dressing, light Italian (1 tablespoon)	0	0	0	0	0
Salmon (3 ounces)	9.84	0.20	0.71	22	0
Salsa (½ cup)	44	0.05	0.16	21	18
Sauerkraut (1 cup)	1.42	0.03	0.18	34	21
Sausage (1 link)	0	0.05	0.01	0.26	0
Shrimp (4 large)	0	0.01	0.03	0.77	0.48
Soft drink with caffeine (12 ounces)	0	0	0	0	0
Soup, cream of chicken (1 cup)	179	0.07	0.07	7	1.24
Soup, tomato (1 cup)	29.28	0.09	0.11	15	66
Soybeans (1 cup cooked)	14	0.47	0.10	200	31
Spaghetti with meatballs (1½ cups)	46	0.38	0.43	101	24
Spareribs (3 ounces)	1.91	0.26	0.22	3	0

VITAMIN E (MG)	CALCIUM (MG)	MAGNESIUM (MG)	POTASSIUM (MG)	SELENIUM (MCG)	ZINC (MG)	CALORIES
15/15	1,000/1,000	420/320	4,700/4,700	55/55	11/8	–
1.40	41	13	207	11	0.66	216
0.70	6	9	186	0.10	0.17	70
.0	12	51	214	2	1	190
.2	15	50	186	2	1	165
0.20	15	12	198	0.17	0.17	100
0.30	6	10	145	0.20	0.12	2
0.36	7	6.46	105	0	0	5
1.78	13	8	76	1	0.20	296
0	117	16	113	13	1	272
2	189	65	548	23	2	170
0	3	5	114	0.30	0.07	40
0	1	11	24	0.80	0.30	31
0.20	6	15	253	14	2	191
0.04	46	38	621	2	0.60	201
0.14	14	36	551	10	0.60	358
4	33	24	256	0.70	1	484
0.21	22	21	88	3	0.50	229
0.30	12	13	350	0.26	0.08	127
0.17	5	4	28	0.04	0.08	10
0.06	20	84	84	19	1	216
0.06	16	19	55	12	0.80	205
0.09	337	19	155	21	1.70	171
0	0	0	2	0.20	0	26
0.95	11	28	475	35	0.60	175
1.53	39	17	275	0.50	0.30	41
0.14	43	18	241	0.90	0.30	45
0.03	1.30	1.56	25	1.87	0.24	125
0	9	7	40	9	0.30	22
0	10	3	3	0.34	0	154
0.25	181	17	272	8	0.67	225
2	12	7	263	0.50	0.24	180
0.02	261	108	970	3	1.64	298
4	138	66	718	39	5	545
0.20	30	15	204	24	3	338

	VITAMIN A (MCG)	VITAMIN B₁ (THIAMIN) (MG)	VITAMIN B₆ (MG)	FOLATE (MCG)	VITAMIN C (MG)
RDA (men/women)	**900/700**	**1.2/1.1**	**1.3/1.3**	**400/400**	**95/75**
Spinach (1 cup)	140	0.02	0.06	58	8
Steak (different cuts)	0	0.10	0.30	6	0
Strawberries (1 cup)	1.66	0.03	0.09	40	97
Submarine sandwich	71	1	0.10	87	12
Sunflower seeds (1/4 cup)	6	0	0.28	82	0.50
Sweet potato (1)	350	0.09	0.25	9	19
Taco salad (1.5 cups)	71	0.10	0.20	83	4
Toaster pastry (1)	148	0.20	0.20	15	0
Tofu (4 ounces)	4.96	0.10	0.06	19	0
Tomato (1 medium)	26	0.02	0.05	9	8
Tuna salad (1 cup)	49	0.06	0.17	16	5
Turkey, skinless (½ breast)	0	0.16	2.26	31	0
Vegetable juice (1 cup)	188	0.10	0.30	51	67
Walnuts (1 cup)	37	0.27	0.70	82	4
Watermelon (1 wedge)	104	0.20	0.40	6	31
Wheat germ (½ cup)	0	0.20	0.40	81	0
Whey protein powder (2 teaspoons)	0	0	0	0	0
Wine, red (3.5 ounces)	0	0	0.03	2	0
Wine, white (3.5 ounces)	0	0	0.01	0	0
Yogurt, low-fat (8 ounces)	2	0.10	0.09	24	1.70

VITAMIN E (MG)	CALCIUM (MG)	MAGNESIUM (MG)	POTASSIUM (MG)	SELENIUM (MCG)	ZINC (MG)	CALORIES
15/15	**1,000/1,000**	**420/320**	**4,700/4,700**	**55/55**	**11/8**	–
0.60	30	24	167	0.30	0.16	10
0.11	4	19	250	12	3.26	217
0.50	27	22	253	1	0.20	46
0	189	68	394	31	2.60	386
12	42	127	248	21.42	1.82	205
1.42	41	27	348	0.30	0.30	103
192	51	416	4	3	0	279
0.90	17	12	57	6.30	0.30	204
0.01	434	37	150	11	1	75
0.33	6	7	146	0	0.11	35
2	35	39	365	84	1	383
0.30	39	109	1,142	95	5	413
12	26	27	467	1	0.50	50
0	73	253	655	21	4.28	654
0.40	41	31	479	0.30	0.20	86
0	27	275	166	91	14	104
0	0	0	260	0	0	21
0	8	13	111	0.20	0.10	88
0	9	10	80	0.20	0.07	86
0	415	37	497	11	1.88	193

A MAN'S PANTRY:
50 BEST FOODS
FOR MEN

5. BEST BROTH
Pacific Natural Foods Low Sodium Organic Free Range Chicken Broth

For better-tasting rice, cook it in this instead of water.

Per cup: 15 calories, 2 g protein, 1 g carbs

10. BEST TERIYAKI SAUCE
Soy Vay Veri Veri Teriyaki

Fueled by real ginger and garlic, it works great as a flavoring for salmon, turkey burgers, or steak.

Per tablespoon: 35 calories, 6 g carbs, 1 g fat

1. BEST BREAD CRUMBS
Wel-Pac Japanese Style Panko

Use this instead of regular bread crumbs to lighten meat loaf and to bread fish.

Per ½ cup: 110 calories, 4 g protein, 20 g carbs (1 g fiber), 1 g fat

6. BEST PEPPER
Simply Organic Black Peppercorns

Pour these whole peppercorns into a grinder, crank, and you'll taste the difference.

0 calories

11. BEST ALL-PURPOSE SPICE
Old Bay 30% Less Sodium Seasoning

Dust this spicy, not-too-salty mix on top of everything from corn to chicken to fish.

0 calories

2. BEST CANOLA OIL
Spectrum Organic Refined Canola Oil

Light, neutral-tasting, and free of genetically modified ingredients.

Per tablespoon: 120 calories, 14 g fat

7. BEST SALT
Diamond Crystal Iodized Salt Sense

These coarse flakes are more intense than table salt, so you can get away with using less.

0 calories

12. BEST SECRET INGREDIENT
McCormick Smoked Paprika

Use a pinch of this Spanish spice to add richness to deviled eggs or chili.

0 calories

3. BEST OLIVE OIL
California Olive Ranch Extra Virgin Olive Oil

This versatile, affordable oil is great for sautéing vegetables or drizzling on mozzarella, or for salad dressings.

Per tablespoon: 120 calories, 14 g fat

8. BEST SOY SAUCE
La Choy Lite

Taste testers liked its light flavor. Use this savory condiment to complement (not overpower) your next stir-fry.

Per tablespoon: 15 calories, 1 g protein, 2 g carbs

13. BEST PRETZEL
Newman's Own Organics High Protein Pretzels

Flour made from peas cranks up the protein content.

Per 22 pretzels: 120 calories, 5 g protein, 22 g carbs (4 g fiber), 2 g fat

4. BEST HOT SAUCE
Frank's RedHot Original Cayenne Pepper Sauce

Our tasters love its slow burn and assertive vinegar kick.

0 calories

9. BEST VINEGAR
Newman's Own Organic Balsamic Vinegar

Mellow and not too sweet, this balsamic ranked as the most balanced in our taste tests. Try it over sliced strawberries.

Per tablespoon: 20 calories, 5 g carbs

14. BEST TORTILLA CHIP
Utz Organic Blue Corn Tortilla Chips

Our tasters said these chips had just the right levels of salt and crunch.

Per ounce: 140 calories, 21 g protein, 19 g carbs (1 g fiber), 3 g fat

15. BEST CRACKER
Back to Nature Organic Stone-ground Wheat Crackers

Great for scooping dips.

Per ½ ounce: 70 calories, 2.5 g protein, 21 g carbs (2 g fiber), 4 g fat

16. BEST POPCORN
Newman's Own Organics Pop's Corn, Light Butter

It has a great flavor, without chemicals.

Per 3½ cups: 112 calories, 3 g protein, 19 g carbs (3.5 g fiber), 3 g fat

17. BEST NUT ALTERNATIVE
Woodstock Organic Pumpkin Seeds

Great for snacking, or add them to a salad of mixed greens.

Per ¼ cup: 180 calories, 9 g protein, 4 g carbs (3 g fiber), 14 g fat

18. BEST NUT
Planter's Men's Health NUT-rition Mix

Did you think any other kind would win? We helped make this stuff!

Per ounce: 170 calories, 6 g protein, 5 g carbs (3 g fiber), 15 g fat

19. BEST BBQ SAUCE
Dinosaur Bar-B-Que Sensuous Slathering Sauce

This sauce has no corn syrup; it does have tomatoes, vinegar, brown sugar, and green pepper.

Per 2 tablespoons: 28 calories, 7 g carbs

20. BEST KETCHUP
Simply Heinz Tomato Ketchup

The bright, flavorful classic we love is now free of corn syrup.

Per tablespoon: 20 calories, 5 g carbs

21. BEST MARINADE
World Harbors Jamaican Style Jerk Marinade and Sauce

The sweet and spicy tropical bite works well with chicken, beef, pork, and even shellfish.

Per tablespoon: 20 calories, 5 g carbs

22. BEST MAYONNAISE
Blue Plate Light Mayonnaise

This mayo has a lemony tang that pumps up the flavors of tuna or turkey sandwiches. And it's lower in calories.

Per tablespoon: 50 calories, 1 g carbs, 5 g fat

23. BEST PEANUT BUTTER
Cream-Nut Natural Peanut Butter

Uniquely smooth and creamy, this jar houses an intense peanut flavor.

Per 2 tablespoons: 190 calories, 8 g protein, 6 g carbs (2 g fiber), 16 g fat

24. BEST MUSTARD
Grey Poupon Country Dijon Mustard

Mustard seeds ratchet up the texture of this blend.

Per tablespoon: 5 calories

25. BEST CANNED TOMATOES
Cento Certified San Marzano Organic Peeled Tomatoes

A rich-tasting Italian variety that doesn't taste like the can.

Per ½ cup: 25 calories, 1 g protein, 5 g carbs (2 g fiber)

26. BEST PICKLE
McClure's Garlic & Dill Spears

Taste one of these snappy, tangy pickles and you won't go back to those yellowish, flavor-free alternatives.

Per ounce: 5 calories, 2 g carbs

27. BEST READY-TO-EAT TUNA
Wild Planet Wild Albacore Tuna

This brand boasts sustainably caught fish with high omega-3 levels and low mercury. Plus it tastes great in a sandwich.

Per 2 ounces: 120 calories, 16 g protein, 6 g fat

28. BEST PROTEIN POWDER
Optimum Nutrition 100% Whey Gold Standard Double Rich Chocolate

A balanced workout-recovery fuel that you'll actually enjoy.

Per scoop: 120 calories, 24 g protein, 3 g carbs, 1 g fat

29. BEST STEEL-CUT OATS
Arrowhead Mills Organic Steel Cut Oats

High in fiber. Great flavor.

Per ¼ cup: 160 calories, 6 g protein, 27 g carbs (8 g fiber), 3 g fat

30. BEST PASTA
Bionaturae Organic Pasta, Whole Wheat Penne Rigate

A satisfying bite and a belly-filling dose of fiber.

Per 2 ounces: 180 calories, 7 g protein, 35 g carbs (6 g fiber), 1.5 g fat

31. BEST QUICK-COOKING RICE
Uncle Ben's Ready Rice Whole Grain Brown

Just nuke it for 90 seconds.

Per cup: 190 calories, 5 g protein, 39 g carbs (3 g fiber), 3 g fat

32. BEST GRAIN
Nature's Earthly Choice Premium Organic Quinoa

This whole grain boasts fiber and complete protein.

Per ¼ cup cooked: 160 calories, 6 g protein, 28 g carbs (3 g fiber), 2.5 g fat

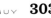

33. BEST FLOUR
King Arthur 100% Organic Unbleached White Whole Wheat

It's amazing for making healthy DIY pizza crust or pasta.

Per ¼ cup: 100 calories, 4 g protein, 22 g carbs (4 g fiber), 0.5 g fat

34. BEST BREAD
Pepperidge Farm Whole Grain 15 Grain

Packed with fiber and protein.

Per slice: 100 calories, 4 g protein, 19 g carbs (3 g fiber), 1 g fat

35. BEST COFFEE BEANS
Starbucks Medium House Blend

These beans yield a cup with a deep but not bitter taste, with a hit of nuttiness on the finish.

0 calories

36. BEST RED WINE UNDER $15
Beronla Rioja Crianza 2008, Spain

The cherry and spice flavors in this smooth, robust red work with everything from chicken to steak.

Per 5 fluid ounces: about 127 calories

37. BEST WHITE WINE UNDER $15
Joel Gott California Sauvignon Blanc 2011

Easy to say, easy to find, easy to enjoy. With flavors of apricot and lemon, this white lights up a meal.

Per 5 fluid ounces: about 128 calories

38. BEST JERKY
Jack Link's Original Beef Jerky

Stash a pack for long drives. The protein will help keep you full on the road.

Per ounce: 80 calories, 15 g protein, 3 g carbs, 1 g fat

39. BEST DRIED FRUIT
Sunsweet D'Noir Preservative Free Prunes

If you need to snack on something sweet, you might as well take in some antioxidants too.

Per 5 prunes: 100 calories, 1 g protein, 24 g carbs (3 g fiber)

40. BEST POTATO CHIP
Boulder Canyon 60% Reduced Sodium Totally Natural Kettle Chips

You won't miss the salt.

Per 14 chips: 140 calories, 2 g protein, 17 g carbs (2 g fiber), 7 g fat

41. BEST SPICY SNACK
Hapi Sriracha Peas

Eat them straight up, or crush them and use as a spicy coating for baked chicken.

Per 28 grams: 120 calories, 4 g protein, 19 g carbs (1 g fiber), 3 g fat

42. BEST GUACAMOLE
Wholly Guacamole Pico de Gallo Style Dip

The pico de gallo adds a slightly spicy salsa kick.

Per 2 tablespoons: 45 calories, 1 g protein, 2 g carbs (1 g fiber), 4 g fat

43. BEST HUMMUS
Athenos Original

Creamy and smooth, with just the right punch of garlic. Try it with carrots and celery.

Per 2 tablespoons: 50 calories, 1 g protein, 5 g carbs (1 g fiber), 3 g fat

44. BEST JAM
Fiordifrutta Strawberry

One of the few organic jams on the market, it's made with wild strawberries and sweetened with apple sugar.

Per tablespoon: 30 calories, 7 g carbs

45. BEST SALAD DRESSING
Newman's Own Lite Honey Mustard Dressing

It works wonders as a marinade for chicken breasts.

Per 2 tablespoons: 70 calories, 7 g carbs, 4 g fat

46. BEST SALSA
Frontera Double Roasted Tomato Salsa

Stir this smoky salsa into a pan of scrambled eggs.

Per 2 tablespoons: 10 calories, 1 g carbs

47. BEST SANDWICH SPREAD
Cento Diced Hot Cherry Peppers

Spice up any sandwich with this chile-packed spread. It's especially good on Italian subs.

Per tablespoon: 5 calories, 1 g carbs

48. BEST STEAK SAUCE
Goodall's Irish Steak Sauce

Enhanced with apples and dates, it adds complexity to meat loaf, burgers, and steaks.

Per tablespoon: 15 calories, 4 g carbs

49. BEST TOMATO SAUCE
Amy's Kitchen Organic Light in Sodium Tomato Basil Sauce

Perfectly sweetened.

Per ½ cup: 90 calories, 2 g protein, 11 g carbs (2 g fiber), 4.5 g fat

50. BEST CANNED BEANS
Eden Foods Organic Garbanzo Beans

Add these fiber-packed, nutty beans to pasta sauce, or toss them into a Greek salad.

Per ½ cup: 130 calories, 7 g protein, 21 g carbs (5 g fiber), 1 g fat

ABOUT THE AUTHORS

Adina Steiman is food and nutrition editor of *Men's Health* magazine and a graduate of Le Cordon Bleu in Paris. She lives in Brooklyn, NY.

Paul Kita is a writer for *Men's Health* magazine and founding editor of the Guy Gourmet blog at Menshealth.com/guy-gourmet. He lives in Allentown, PA.

INDEX

Underscored page references indicate boxed text. **Boldfaced** page references indicate photographs.

E

F